Clinical Mechanics in the Gut
An Introduction

Authored by

Hans Gregersen

College of Bioengineering
Chongqing University
Chongqing
China

&

James Christensen

University of Iowa Hospitals and Clinics
Iowa City
USA

CONTENTS

FOREWORD

Bioengineering and biomechanics have impacted on orthopedics and cardiovascular science for years for the benefit of basic scientists, developers, health care personnel and patients. However, it never gained widespread impact in gastroenterology. There may be many reasons for the lack of use of bioengineering principles and biomechanics theory in gastroenterology, some may relate to ignorance and lack of recognition, others to difficulties changing the way of thinking. This is about to change and the book entitled Biomechanics of the Gastrointestinal Tract from 2002 by Hans Gregersen and the present book on clinical biomechanics in gastroenterology by Gregersen and Christensen will certainly change this.

Bioengineering in its present concept was introduced by Professor YC Fung from University of California San Diego more than 40 years ago and Professor Fung is truly considered one of the founding notabilities of bioengineering and the father of modern biomechanics. Fung authored several books on continuum mechanics and biomechanics, and he tutored many students including Hans Gregersen, one of the authors of this book, and myself. Good ideas spread with the wind which certainly has been the case with Fung´s ideas. The present book is an example of how basic bioengineering principles can be used to change the look on gastrointestinal diseases. I sincerely hope that the ideas and concepts in this book will spread and that bioengineering principles will come into the mind of gastroenterologists.

Zhuang Fengyuan
Department of Bioengineering (Now School of
Bioscience and Medical Engineering)
Beihang University
School of Life Science
Beijing Institute of Technology
China
International Academy of Astronautics
France

PREFACE

All multicellular animals move fluids through themselves and move themselves through fluids. Evolution has created the most appropriate conceivable means for organisms to deal with the movements of fluids internally and externally.

In animals, the management of fluids encompasses the flows that exist in internal organ systems. For most people, the cardiovascular system first comes to mind when they think about fluid mechanics in biological organ systems. Also, when they consider the alimentary tract, most physiologists think first of the biochemical processes involved in digestion and absorption rather than the mechanics. The fact that the gastrointestinal tract is basically a mechanical device should be so evident as to require no comment. Often, however, both the science and the practice of gastroenterology seem to disregard that insight. Walter B. Cannon's book on gastrointestinal mechanics, published in 1911, did little, in retrospect, to foster much further reflection about the gut as a machine. Also, the renewed dialog in both the laboratory and the clinic about gastrointestinal motility has not generally employed the perspectives of the engineer, the principles of physics and the tools of the mathematician.

Even though the gastrointestinal tract constitutes a much more complex biohydraulic system than the cardiovascular system, much less attention has gone to its mechanical operations. But mechanical operations are primary in the digestive system. The physical treatment of materials, including their conveyance from one place to another, must precede their chemical treatments, digestion and absorption.

Gastrointestinal motility, the familiar term used to refer to the mechanical behavior of the alimentary tract, actually encompasses three different and related operations:

- the active wall movements that initiate the shift of the fluid contents,
- the functions within the systems that regulate the active wall movements,
- the flows that the active wall movements produce.

Confusingly, the term, "motility" is used sometimes for the whole operation and sometimes for one or another of these three component processes alone. For that reason, we have used "mechanics" in the title of this book because that term seems to us to indicate our emphasis.

The gastrointestinal tract constitutes a series of motor organs, each with its own pattern of motions and set of controlling mechanisms, and each serving as both conduit and pump. Each organ exhibits rostrocaudal polarity in function and, because the organs are linked "nose-to-tail" (except for the gallbladder), each one prepares the fluid it receives to make it suitable for treatment by the following organ.

Animals need such a system of alimentary pumps and conduits in order to meet several needs:

- to regulate the forward flow of nutrient-containing ingested substances

- to enhance the enzymatic degradation that releases the nutrients from food
- to optimize the extraction of the nutrients from the degraded materials
- to control the disposition of the undigested residue

Each kind of pump in the tract induces the specific pattern of flow required for the particular function of each part. At different places along the tract, these pumps provide different flow patterns to meet these nutritional requirements. These constitute antegrade flows, retrograde flows, laminar mixing flows and storage. Despite the different behaviors of the various organs, however, all parts of the gastrointestinal tract in all animals operate on the basis of fundamentally identical structures and systems. The organs differ from one another mainly quantitatively, in the degree to which they use one or another variation in the mechanism.

To the engineer, the gastrointestinal tract presents a machine of extraordinary intricacy, one that refuses to remain stable. Its non-Newtonian fluids vary constantly and widely in physical properties as they move along the tract. The motions of the several organs vary continuously in both quality and quantity. Self-regulation differently characterizes each organ as well as in the system as a whole. This complexity gives the alimentary tract an adaptability that allows animals to use a wide variety of substrates having very different physical characteristics as a source of the energy needed to sustain life.

This complex mechanical system, the alimentary canal long waited to be illuminated by the science of mechanics but biologists, lacking appropriate training, could not do the job. Now, however, a new discipline, bioengineering, promises to bring the concepts of engineering to the analysis of mechanical processes in all biological systems. Bioengineering, which has grown tremendously in the past decade, has found its most ready application in the examination of musculoskeletal mechanics and cardiovascular function.

The alimentary canal remains almost untouched by bioengineers, but not entirely so. Some work in recent years has provided glimpses into the details of the flows of gastrointestinal fluids, hints about the kinds of motions that occur in the muscular walls of the tract, and clues about the regulating mechanisms. These advances have paved the way to a fuller examination of the tract as the mechanical device that it is, employing the perspective of the engineer as well as that of the descriptive biologist. This book attempts to introduce this fundamental change in outlook, to establish a new point of view about this biomechanical system.

In respect to the practice of medicine, current concepts in gastrointestinal motor function continue to rest largely on empirical grounds, and the mechanical operation of the gut under various conditions remains hard to predict.

The great problem in this area of study remains the gulf that separates biology from the physical sciences. Many biologists lack appropriate understanding of the physical sciences, while physical scientists generally fail to comprehend the complicated nature of gastrointestinal anatomy, flows, and forces. Greater shared understanding between biologists and physical scientists must contribute to the better management of the many clinical disorders of this biohydraulic system. It could also lead to the design of better mechanical devices to transport fluids in the wider world.

By publishing this book, we hope to advance biomechanics and bioengineering in the thinking of both investigators and practitioners in gastrointestinal science. It builds on top of the book Biomechanics of the Gastrointestinal Tract by Gregersen from 2002 that had a focus on the basic science aspects of gastrointestinal biomechanics. We believe that the established methods and concepts of physical science will provide the framework for a keener understanding of the mechanics of the gut than we now have.

ACKNOWLEDGEMENTS

We wish to acknowledge many coworkers, collaborators and students who conducted some of the research the book is based on and who kindly provided some of the figures and materials published in this book. Personal assistant Wu Min (Ivy) is kindly thanked for her editing of the text and figures we also thank funding agencies from China, USA and Denmark for support.

CONFLICT OF INTEREST

The authors confirm that this ebook contents have no conflict of interest.

Hans Gregersen
College of Bioengineering
Chongqing University
Chongqing
China

&

James Christensen
University of Iowa Hospitals and Clinics
Iowa City
USA

Clinical Mechanics in the Gut
An Introduction

CHAPTER 1

The Geometry of the System: The Structure of the Gastrointestinal Tract as a Mechanical Device

Abstract: The gastrointestinal tract constitutes an uninterrupted channel through the organism with separate ports for intake and output. This chapter deals first with the basic structure of the wall of the alimentary conduit and with the modifications encountered in each of the various organs, with emphasis on basis anatomy and morphology of the system for a better understanding of the mechanical (motility, distensibility and flow) function and mechanosensory function.

Keywords: Anatomy, esophagus, gastrointestinal tract, large intestine, small intestine, sphincters, stomach, structure.

1.1. INTRODUCTION

The gastrointestinal tract constitutes an uninterrupted channel through the organism with separate ports for intake and output. The entrance port lies at the cephalic (or rostral) end of the animal and the exit port is found at the caudal extremity. Although the tract functions as a single pathway, it really constitutes a series of regions, the component organs of the tract (Fig. **1**).

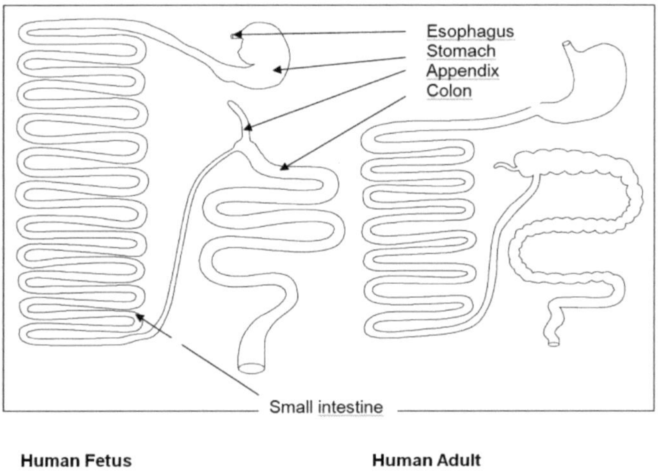

Figure 1: Diagram of the fetal and adult human gastrointestinal tract. It is drawn so to show the shapes and continuity of the various organs and parts and their proportionate dimensions. In both drawings, the esophagus is amputated: it extends through the thorax for approximately the length of the stomach.

Hans Gregersen and James Christensen

Each of these parts serves a different set of needs in animal nutrition but they all participate in the net transfer of material in the rostrocaudal direction.

Even though the distinctive names of these organs suggest that they are distinct and separate structures, they actually resemble one another in their fundamental makeup. Each of them exhibits variations on a basic plan. Their structural modifications correlate to their special mechanical operations. Thus, the esophagus transfers swallowed matter to the stomach, and the stomach serves to retain material and to deliver it slowly to the intestine. The small and large intestines must create patterns of flow in intraluminal fluids that assure the efficient extraction of water and nutrient substances.

The geometry described here applies to all higher animals. Animals occupy different ecological niches. They vary accordingly in diet and the structure of the gastrointestinal motor apparatus varies correspondingly. The generic description given here applies to man of course, and human specializations are pointed out appropriately.

This chapter deals first with the basic structure of the wall of the alimentary conduit and then with the modifications encountered in each of the various organs. In accordance with convention, this discussion of gastrointestinal anatomy excludes the mouth, dealing only with the pharynx and the following parts of the system. The reader is referred to general textbooks for further reading on the anatomy of the gastrointestinal tract. In addition references [1-13] are very informative.

1.2. THE GENERAL SCHEME

The wall of the gastrointestinal tract is a laminar structure (Fig. **2**). Its various layers necessarily operate mechanically as a unit because they are bound together. However, the layers differ from one another in that they possess dissimilar properties, both physical and physiological. Thus, they contribute differently to the mechanical function of the system. These layers constitute layers of tissues of different kinds: muscle, connective tissue, nerves, and epithelium.

The muscle layers generate forces that distort the cylindrical conduit as they contract. The wall movements shift or propel the luminal contents appropriately. The connective tissue layers (as well as muscle when not contracted) provide a framework that determines the passive physical properties of the gut wall. The layers composed of nerves provide the controls that govern the spatiotemporal distribution of contractions. The epithelial layer that covers the luminal surface transfers dissolved substances from the gut lumen into the blood circulation.

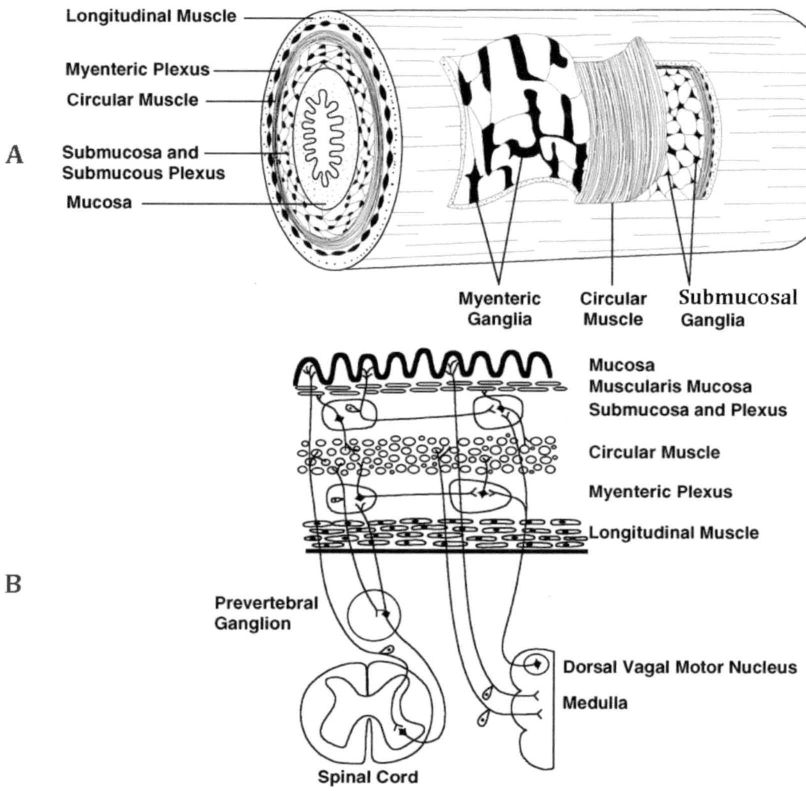

Figure 2: Diagrams to show the various layers of the gastrointestinal wall and their components. **A**) is a cutaway to show especially the positions of the two plexuses of nerves. **B**) is a diagram showing the hypothetical interconnections of the two plexuses.

Gastrointestinal muscle is visceral muscle, also called involuntary muscle because its behavior is independent of the will. This variety of muscle also constitutes the muscular wall in other internal organs, the blood vessels and the motile viscera of the genital and urinary tracts. It is also called "smooth" muscle because of the uniformity of its appearance under the light microscope.

There is one exception to the general rule that gastrointestinal muscle is visceral muscle. In the most cephalic part of the tract, the pharynx and the rostral part of the esophagus, the muscle is striated (or somatic) muscle, like the muscle of the musculoskeletal system. This variety of muscle is also called voluntary muscle because its operation is generally regulated by the will.

Gastrointestinal connective tissue makes up most of the thickness of the submucosa and the mucosa and a large part of the muscle layers. It consists of fibers of collagen and elastin, together with fibroblasts and other small cells. As in other parts of the body, the kind and the density of the fibrous components vary to supply the mechanical characteristics that the locus requires.

Gastrointestinal nerves form a complex nervous system within the wall of the gut, the enteric nervous system. This system operates in considerable independence of the central nervous system. It contains a variety of kinds of nerve cells. They give off axons (the efferent processes of nerve cells, those that convey signals away from the nerve cell body) that are devoid of a myelin sheath. The myelin sheath is a coating that surrounds many axons in the central nervous system and thereby gives to them the ability to transmit nerve impulses very rapidly. The absence of myelin in the enteric nerves implies that there is no need in the gut for the very rapid transmission of the nerve impulse.

The epithelial layer that lines the tract also varies from one organ to another to serve the general function of each part. Thus, in the esophagus it mainly protects the deeper layers of the organ from noxious substances that may come into the lumen. In the stomach, it elaborates the gastric juice. In the intestines it extracts water and nutrient substances from the luminal contents.

The gut wall requires a rich blood supply both to provide the chemical environment necessary for the normal operation of all its different kinds of cells and to take up absorbed nutrients. The arteries and veins, traveling together, penetrate the main muscle layer as relatively large vessels and then branch between and within the inner layers of the wall. Their points of penetration form widely separated weak points in the major muscle coat but these discontinuities seem to have little effect on gastrointestinal mechanics.

1.2.1. The Muscle Layers and Their Composition

1.2.1.1. The Main Muscle Coat

The principal muscle coat of the gut (also called the muscularis propria) constitutes two separate layers. In each layer, a network of collagen fibers forms the basic structure that defines the gross geometry of the sheet. This structure is termed the *stroma* (from the Latin word for a bed covering). Within the interstices of this web lie the muscle cells, tightly attached both to one another (Fig. **3**) and to the fibrous elements of the mesh.

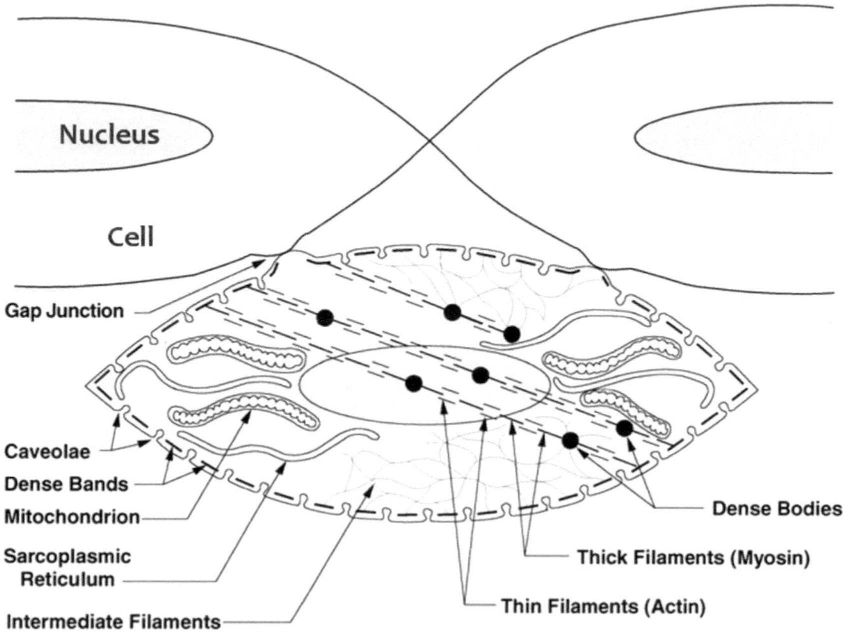

Figure 3: A diagram of a smooth muscle cell to show its internal structure and its connection to other such cells. Collagen stroma, not shown, fills the space between the muscle cells.

The muscle cells themselves are commonly described as spindle-shaped or fusiform, but that is the general form they have only when they are examined in their most elongated conformation, which is never achieved in life. Although they change shape as they move, they can be viewed as generally cylindrical, each cell being capable of shortening separately in the process of contraction.

In each of the principal muscle layers of the gut, the muscle cells all lie with their axes essentially parallel. Their common attachment to the connective tissue stroma integrates their separate actions. Since all the muscle cells within a field usually contract and relax essentially simultaneously or in a coordinated pattern, the whole layer of muscle cells appears to move as a unit. Since each cell is only a few hundred microns long, even a small contraction of the muscle involves many thousands of cells acting together.

The two layers of muscle in the main muscle coat differ in the alignment of their muscle cells. The cells in the outer layer of the muscularis propria are oriented with their axes in the direction of the axis of the cylindrical conduit. Therefore, this layer is called the longitudinal muscle layer. In the inner layer of muscle, the axes of the cells lie in the direction of the circumference of the conduit. For this reason, this layer is called the circular muscle layer.

Only about half the volume of a mass of gastrointestinal muscle is intracellular volume and most of that represents the interior space of muscle cells. The extracellular space constitutes principally extracellular water and the network of the collagen and elastin fibers that forms the connective tissue stroma.

A small proportion of space in the muscle is occupied by other cellular structures. In the longitudinal muscle layer, these are principally the axons that ramify among the muscle cells and the cellular structures that make up the infrequent capillaries. The proportion of space occupied by such non-muscular components is trivial from the mechanical point of view.

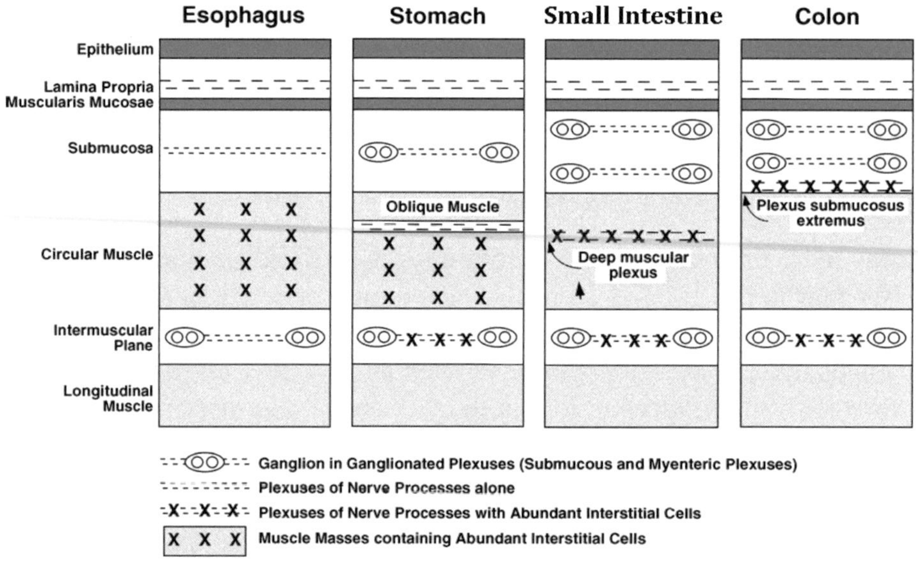

Figure 4: A diagram of the principal planes of concentration of interstitial cells of Cajal in relation to the circular muscle layer in the various organs. Organs vary in the exact position of the planes of interstitial cells, which are marked as "X"s.

The circular muscle layer contains a special set of modified muscle cells, the interstitial cells of Cajal (Fig. **4**) that constitute only a small fraction of the total number of cells, probably less than five percent. These stellate cells give out long processes that extend widely to contact many muscle cells. The interstitial cells in the circular muscle layer possess an intimate relationship with the axons that regulate the operation of the muscle, seemingly being interposed between axons and muscle cells. Axons also contact muscle cells directly. The interstitial cells are akin to muscle cells, derived from the same ancestral cells but modified in form probably in such a way as to provide especially for the transmission of information between nerve and muscle and between muscle cells within the muscle mass.

1.2.1.2. The Muscle of the Mucosa

A third layer of muscle occurs throughout almost the entire tract, the muscle of the mucosa (muscularis mucosae). The submucosa separates it from the main muscle coat. The general structure of the mucosal muscle is the same as that of the other muscle layers, a collagen mesh forming a stroma that surrounds the muscle cells and attaches to them. The muscle cells are generally arranged with their axes lying in many directions with reference to the axis of the cylinder in the tract. It forms one layer of the mucosa, the deepest layer. The other two layers are the lamina propria, a thin sheet of connective tissue, and the epithelium, the layer of cells that lines the lumen

1.2.2. The Connective Tissue Layers and Their Composition

Connective tissue, like that found throughout the animal body, serves in the gut especially to provide the passive mechanical properties of the organs. It constitutes principally collagen fibers forming a loose and apparently unorganized mesh. Special studies, however, show them to have a clear organization, forming skeletons for the several layers of the wall.

There are several different kinds of collagen, distinguished in the molecular structure of the fiber, and these have slightly different physical properties. These collagen fibers lie among the muscle cells in the muscular layers. Differences in the passive physical properties of the various layers could reflect differences in the proportions of the various types of collagen present, in the precise geometry of the collagen network, and in the proportion of the whole mass that constitutes collagen. Connective tissue also contains other kinds of cells that serve immune or other non-mechanical functions.

1.2.2.1. The Submucosa

In most gastrointestinal organs, the submucosa lies between the main muscle coat and the mucosa. This is a broad layer that makes up a large proportion of the wall, nearly half in the esophagus, but much less in the intestine. Quantitatively, it consists principally of connective tissue but it also contains many kinds of small cells with general maintenance and immune functions. Most of the submucosa, however, is open space occupied by water. Because of its thickness and structural laxity, this layer of the gut wall allows the mucosa to move easily and widely over the inner surface of the main muscle coat. The submucosa also contains the network of nerves called the submucosal plexus and the small blood vessels that supply the mucosa.

1.2.2.2. The Subserosa

A layer of epithelial cells, the serosa, covers the main muscle coat on the outside. The serosa is a membrane that envelops the whole of the intraabdominal gastrointestinal tract. It is continuous with the peritoneum, the lining of the abdomen. This serosal epithelium is tightly attached to the outer (longitudinal) muscle layer by the subserosa, a thin and dense layer of collagen fibers. The subserosa contains also a small number of nerve fibers.

1.2.2.3. The Lamina Propria

Another layer of connective tissue, the lamina propria, lies between the mucosal muscle layer and the gastrointestinal epithelium, the layer of cells that lines the lumen of the entire gastrointestinal tract. The lamina propria is somewhat denser in its composition than the submucosa. Fibers of collagen and elastin, lacking any obvious organization, constitute the principal matrix elements in this layer. The layer also contains many kinds of scattered small cells that act in immune function and in general maintenance function, as well as a few nerve fibers. It firmly joins the epithelium to the mucosal muscle.

1.2.2.4. The Intermuscular Space

The myenteric plexus occupies the space between the two layers of the main muscle coat. This plexus is embedded in a thin lamina of connective tissue that contains a scattering of other types of cells. Interstitial cells of Cajal form a network within the plane of the myenteric plexus in most regions, but not all.

1.2.3. The Epithelial Layers and their Composition

1.2.3.1. The Gastrointestinal Epithelium

The gastrointestinal epithelium covers the innermost surface of the gastrointestinal tract. This layer of cells differs greatly in structure and function in the various parts of the tract. The epithelial cells are closely attached to one another through intercellular junctions to form a continuous and quite homogeneous sheet. These junctions serve an important mechanical function by sealing off the luminal space. The junctions are, however, fragile structures that cannot provide much physical strength to the epithelium as a membrane. That arises more from the adherence of the epithelial cells to the basal lamina, a thin sheet of amorphous material that lies between the epithelial cells and the lamina propria. The fragile epithelial cells are mounted, as it were, on a comparatively tough sheet. The mechanical properties of the basal lamina remain unknown.

1.2.3.2. The Serosa

The serosa, a sheet of epithelial cells that encloses the intraabdominal parts of the gastrointestinal tract in the abdominal cavity, is continuous with the identical membrane that lines the abdominal cavity. This membrane constitutes a single structure, called the serosa where it encloses the gut and called the peritoneum where it lines the cavity within which most of the gut lies. Its cells are adherent to one another other directly and through their position on the collagen mesh of the subserosa (see 1.2.2.2.). They secrete a fluid that lubricates the outer surface of the parts of the gastrointestinal tract that lie in the peritoneal cavity. This allows low friction movement of the loops of gut that are compacted within the abdominal cavity.

1.2.4. Intramural Nerves

A system of nerves extends throughout all layers of the gastrointestinal wall. Its operation is most conspicuously expressed in the motions of the muscular walls, although it also serves other functions, such as the regulation of secretion and absorption. It is usually thought of, however, principally in terms of its regulation of muscular contractions and relaxations in all three layers of muscle. Because of the conspicuous sensitivity of the motions of the walls of the alimentary canal to mechanical influences, this intramural system of nerves must include elements with the ability to sense motion in the wall of the gut. These receptors are yet not well characterized from a mechanical point of view. There seem to be chemoreceptors in the gut wall as well, nervous structures that detect changes in the chemical nature of the luminal content. Like mechanoreceptors, these receptors are yet not well characterized.

1.2.4.1. The Myenteric Plexus

The loose collagen matrix in the cleft between the two layers of the main muscle coat, the intermuscular plane, contains a particularly dense network of nerves, the myenteric plexus. This set of nerves is essential to the regulation of the contractions of the two adjacent muscle layers. The basic form of the nerve cells in this plexus, a single rounded cell body that gives off one or more long processes called axons, gives this network its structure (Fig. **5**).

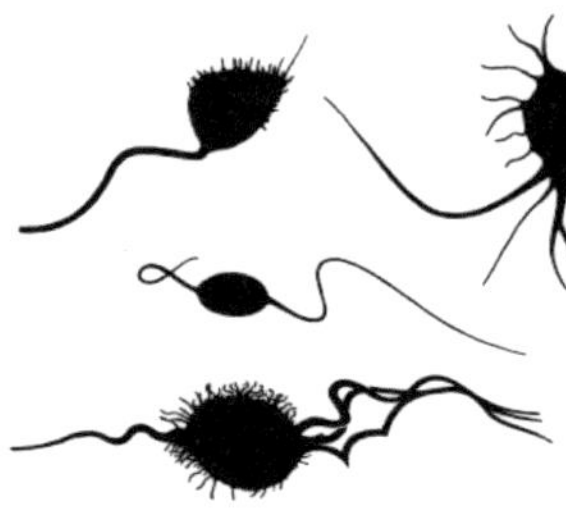

Figure 5: A diagram of various shapes of nerve cells showing the characteristic short dendrites and long axons. The functional implications of the different shapes remain to be discovered.

The bodies of the nerve cell form clusters or nodes, the ganglia. Bundles of axons connect ganglia together to make a two-dimensional rhomboidal mesh (Fig. **6**). The nodes in this network are the ganglia, clusters of nerve cell bodies, while the cords are bundles of axons, nerve processes that conduct impulses away from nerve cells.

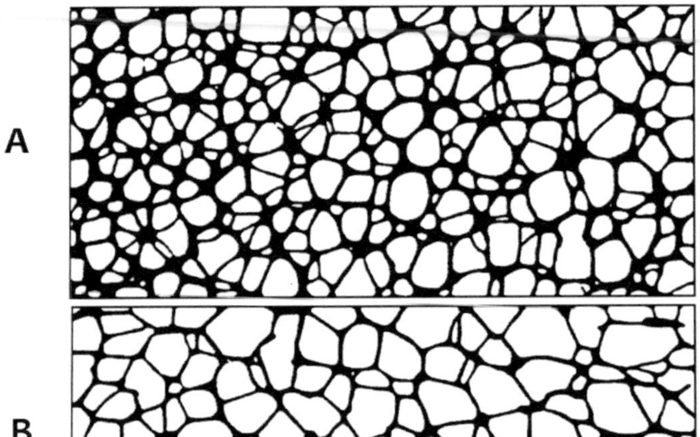

Figure 6: Silhouette drawings of the myenteric plexus as traced from the colon (A) and the rectum (B) of the guinea pig. This illustrates the variation possible in the geometry of the myenteric plexus.

The motions of the gastrointestinal wall might stretch or break the axons without the safeguard provided by the geometry of the myenteric plexus. The mesh can be considerably deformed without damage because its polygonal structure can accommodate great change in either the axial or the circumferential direction so long as a change in one dimension is compensated by a change in the other. Also, the whole plexus floats in the loose collagen stroma of the intermuscular space.

Three functional categories of nerve cells (neurons) make up the myenteric plexus. They cannot be distinguished in geometric terms. They constitute:

- cells that pick up information from the gut wall (sensory neurons),
- cells that carry information directly to muscle or to other effector cells (motor neurons),
- cells that connect sensory to motor nerve cells (internuncial neurons).

Mechanoreceptors essential to the self-regulatory function of the gastrointestinal musculature must be present within the gastrointestinal wall. In at least two places, the esophagus and the rostral part of the stomach, special structures, the intraganglionic laminar endings (IGLE's) of the myenteric plexus ganglia (Fig. 7) have been proposed as mechanoreceptors.

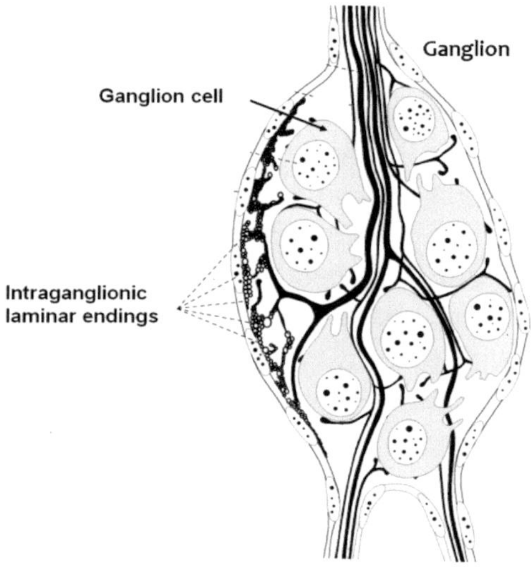

Figure 7: A diagram of the intraganglionic laminar endings in a ganglion of the esophageal myenteric plexus. They lie at the periphery of the ganglion. Morphological evidence indicates that these structures are vagal (parasympathetic) mechanoreceptors.

1.2.4.2. The Submucosal Plexus

The thick and gelatinous submucosa contains a network of nerves that resembles the myenteric plexus. This submucosal plexus regulates the whole mucosa, especially the mucosal muscle, as well as, in some places at least, the circular muscle layer of the muscularis propria. Its ganglia and interconnecting nerve bundles, however, are much less densely distributed than those of the myenteric plexus and the mesh they form has a less uniform polygonal pattern. The geometry of the submucosal plexus seems, similarly, to protect it from mechanical damage that might ensue from the motions of the muscular wall of the gastrointestinal tract.

1.2.4.3. The Nerves of the Lamina Propria

The lamina propria contains nerve processes connecting the submucosal plexus to the epithelium. For the most part, these fibers seem to extend mainly in the z-axis of the cylinder, perpendicular to the luminal surface, passing only a short distance in the axial and circumferential directions. They follow a convoluted track, accommodating themselves to the motions of the mucosa.

1.2.4.4. The Nerves of the Serosa

The serosa contains mechanoreceptive neural structures, the Pacinian corpuscles like those of the skin. They are the endings of sensory nerves but there seems to be little more information about them in the serosa.

1.2.5. Extramural Nerves

Despite the autonomy of the intramural nervous system in the gut (which justifies its common portrayal as a “little brain”), it must interact to some extent with regulatory centers in the brain and spinal cord. Major nerve trunks connect the gastrointestinal tract with the central nervous system (Fig. **8**), forming two separate sets of such extramural connections, the craniosacral and thoracolumbar systems. Both systems contain both motor and sensory pathways, respectively carrying nerve traffic toward and away from the gut. The two systems function separately. forming two separate sets of such extramural connections, the craniosacral and thoracolumbar systems. Both systems contain both motor and sensory pathways, respectively carrying nerve traffic toward and away from the gut. The two systems function separately.

The two terms, craniosacral and thoracolumbar, designate the anatomic arrangement of the extramural nerves. They are also commonly called sympathetic (thoracolumbar) and parasympathetic (craniosacral) connections.

These latter two terms reflect the function of the two pathways as components of the autonomic nervous system. Together, these two components make up the autonomic nervous system, the system of nerves connecting the brain and the spinal cord to all visceral structures, including the gut.

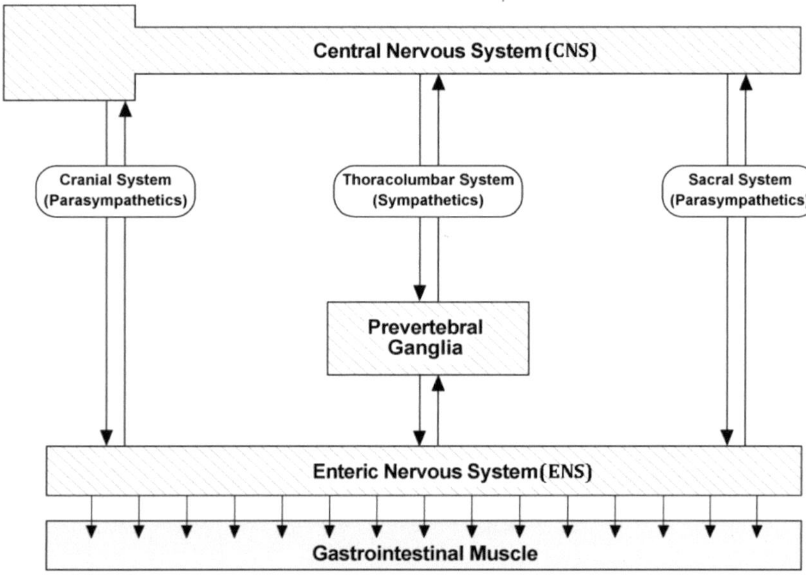

Figure 8: A diagram of the relationship between the central nervous system and the enteric nervous system and their connections by way of the extrinsic innervation of the gut.

1.2.5.1. The Craniosacral Innervation

The craniosacral innervation links the gastrointestinal tract to the two parts of the central nervous system, the brainstem in the cranial part of the central nervous system and the sacral part of the spinal cord. The cranial component of the innervation constitutes the tenth cranial (vagus) nerves, joining the gastrointestinal tract to the sensory and motor centers of that cranial nerve in the region of the fourth ventricle of the brain. The sacral part passes through the pelvic nerves that arise from the sacral roots of those nerves.

In the gut, the distribution of the fibers from the vagus nerves extends from the rostral end of the esophagus, to the midportion of the large intestine. The peripheral distribution of the sacral portion extends from the middle of the large intestine to the caudal extremity of the tract. The two distributions may overlap to some degree.

Nerve fibers from the craniosacral innervation mainly contact intramural neurons within the myenteric plexus. Their distributions vary among organs, as discussed later.

1.2.5.2. The Thoracolumbar Innervation

The thoracolumbar innervation connects the gastrointestinal tract to the thoracic and lumbar segments of the spinal cord. These fibers, passing through the splanchnic nerves which are formed by the fusion of the segmental nerves that emanate from the thoracic part of the spinal cord, extend to the prevertebral (or retroperitoneal) ganglia, clusters of nerve cell bodies. The nerve fibers that originate in the thoracolumbar part of the spinal cord terminate here in synapse with nerve call bodies from which nerve fibers extend alongside the arterial blood supply to the gastrointestinal wall where they end in the myenteric plexus and in small arteries.

A complete nerve pathway in the thoracolumbar system contains two neurons, one cell body lying in the spinal cord and the other in a prevertebral ganglion. Thus, the prevertebral ganglia provide a stage for sensorimotor integration outside both the central and the enteric nervous systems. This appears to be important in the transfer of information over long distances along the alimentary tract.

1.3. THE SPECIALIZED GEOMETRY CHARACTERISTICS OF THE ORGANS

1.3.1. Pharynx and Pharyngoesophageal Sphincter

1.3.1.1. Musculature

The pharyngeal musculature differs greatly from the general scheme. There is no mucosal muscle. The muscularis propria consists entirely of striated (somatic) muscle cells and the direction of their axes is exclusively circumferential rather that axial. Thus, the pharyngeal muscularis propria constitutes only one layer, a circular muscle layer.

Three distinct somatic muscles encircle the lumen to form the wall of the pharynx. These are the superior, middle and inferior pharyngeal constrictors. They overlap one another to encase the whole pharynx. Each constrictor constitutes two parts, right and left. The halves are physically continuous, fused at the midline so that each constrictor acts as a single encircling unit.

The inferior constrictor thickens at the junction of the pharynx to the esophagus to form the pharyngoesophageal sphincter, or cricopharyngeus muscle (Fig. **9**).

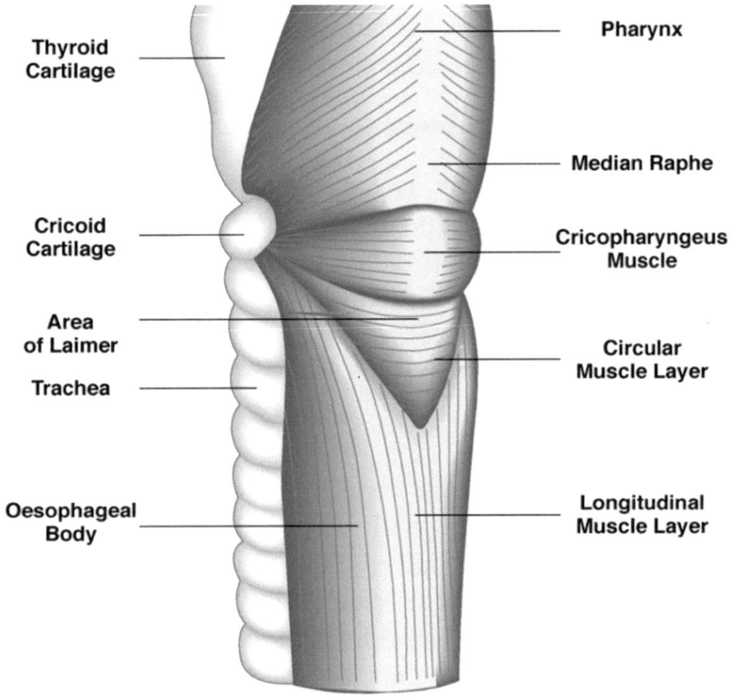

Figure 9: A posterior oblique view of the pharynx and rostral end of the esophagus to show the relationship of the cricopharyngeus muscle (upper esophageal or pharyngoesophageal sphincter) to adjacent structures.

Although this sphincter is continuous with the pharyngeal musculature, it is distinguishable in its greater thickness and in its gross anatomical relationship to the airway. Instead of encircling the pharynx like the rest of the pharyngeal constrictors, the sphincter muscle is attached at both ends to the ends of the cricoid cartilage. Thus, its contraction closes the lumen by compression of the pharyngoesophageal junction against the trachea, whereas the pharyngeal constrictors close the lumen by circumferential occlusion.

1.3.1.2. Connective Tissue

The pharynx is covered on the outside by a collagenous sheath that separates it from other structures in the neck. This allows the muscular organ to move without significant tethering. The very loose collagen attachment between the pharynx and adjacent structures does not influence the movements of the pharyngeal musculature.

There is a similar sheath of connective tissue between the overlapping constrictors themselves that allows them to move a little over one another. Such a connective tissue sheath also covers the luminal surface of the musculature to form a base for the attachment of the epithelium. There are no layers corresponding to the submucosa and lamina propria that characterize the rest of the gut.

1.3.1.3. Epithelium

The epithelium lining the pharynx is squamous epithelium, like the skin but devoid of the relatively tough keratinized outer layer that characterizes the skin. As a squamous epithelium, it is tougher and less permeable than the epithelium of the more caudal parts of the gastrointestinal tract.

There is no serosa surrounding the pharynx because it does not lie within a serosal cavity.

1.3.1.4. Intramural Nerves

The nerves in the pharyngeal wall are the terminal branches of the glossopharyngeal nerve, which supplies this striated musculature. Their motor nerve processes terminate as motor end plates, the classical neuromuscular junctions of somatic nerves and muscles. Somatic sensory nerve fibers in the pharynx end in muscle spindles, mechanoreceptors that appear to be identical to those found in somatic muscle elsewhere. Thus, this musculature functions as a striated or somatic muscle.

The sensory innervation of the mucosa is sympathetic.

1.3.1.5. Extrinsic Nerves

Branches of the glossopharyngeal nerve provide the motor and sensory supply to the muscles of the pharynx, including the pharyngoesophageal sphincter. These pass directly between the pharynx and the nuclei of that nerve in the brain stem near the fourth ventricle.

1.3.2. Esophagus and Esophagogastric Sphincter

1.3.2.1. Musculature

The muscle of the esophagus differs from the general scheme principally in the nature of the muscle cells. In man, from the rostral end of the organ, at the pharyngoesophageal junction, to a point about one-third of the way to the stomach, the musculature is striated (somatic) muscle, like that of the pharynx. At that level, the muscle becomes visceral (smooth) muscle, which makes up the muscle throughout the remainder of the gastrointestinal tract. The two kinds of muscle cells, striated and smooth (or somatic and visceral), are intermingled in the middle of the esophagus for only a very short distance within both main muscle layers. A slight thickening of the inner (circular) muscle layer in the last centimeter above the stomach characterizes the esophagogastric (lower esophageal) sphincter.

The interstitial cells of Cajal in the circular smooth muscle layer are distributed diffusely throughout the thickness of that layer. There are none in the striated muscle of the rostral part of the organ.

The muscle of the mucosa in the esophagus differs from the general scheme in two ways. It is very thick, fully as thick as the inner layer of the main muscle coat, and its cylindrical muscle fibers (visceral muscle throughout the whole organ) all lie with their axes parallel to the axis of the esophagus. This implies that the contraction of the mucosal muscle layer tends to shorten the esophagus, like the contractions of the outer (longitudinal) muscle layer of the main muscle coat.

1.3.2.2. Connective Tissue

The esophagus possesses a special connective tissue structure in the form of the phrenoesophageal ligament, a grommet-like collar made of collagen and elastin fibers that seals the organ within the opening in the diaphragm through which the organ passes, the esophageal hiatus. This ligament has two leaflets or layers, one that inserts on the circumference of the esophagus at about the rostral edge of the esophagogastric sphincter and one that inserts similarly at about the caudal border of the sphincter (Fig. **10**).

The phrenoesophageal ligament is extensive and elastic enough to allow the considerable axial movement of the esophagus through the diaphragm that must occur in breathing and swallowing. Since the rostral end of the organ is tethered to the cricoid cartilage, this ligamentous attachment to the diaphragm maintains the esophagus in its rostrocaudal orientation throughout the excursions that result from movements of the body, the diaphragm and the stomach.

1.3.2.3. Epithelium

The esophageal epithelium, like that of the pharynx, is a non-keratinized squamous epithelium. As such, it is relatively tough and impermeable. It ends almost exactly at the point where the musculature of the esophagus joins that of the stomach. In other words, the very different epithelia of the esophagus and stomach are strictly confined to their respective organs in normal circumstances. In a common disease state, chronic gastroesophageal reflux, the epithelial junction often lies well above the junction of the two organs.

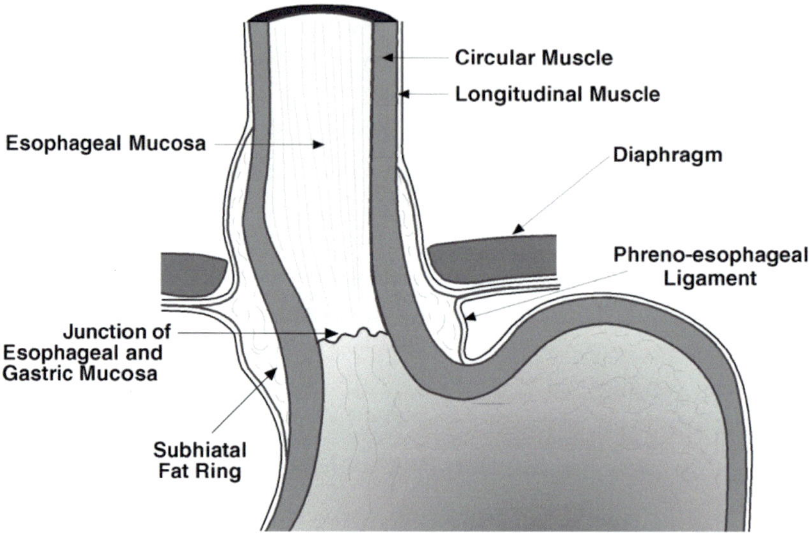

Figure 10: A diagram of the phrenoesophageal ligament and the other features of the esophagogastric junction.

1.3.2.4. Intramural Nerves

The myenteric plexus of the esophagus differs from the general scheme in its relative paucity of ganglia and in its lack of a regular polygonal pattern. The interganglionic bundles of axons extend mainly in the direction of the axis of the organ. Many large nerve bundles, branches from the tenth (vagus) nerves, run through the plexus parallel to the axis of the organ. The fact that axial elongation of the esophagus does not occur in its normal operation allows the presence of these axially oriented bundles of nerve fibers in the wall of the esophagus. Otherwise, they would be stretched or broken.

The submucosal plexus in the esophagus also differs from the general scheme. There are no ganglia. The few nerve fiber bundles to be found in the submucosa contain axons that extend there from the myenteric plexus or the extrinsic nerves.

A comparatively simple network of axons (arising from the submucosal plexus) in the lamina propria gives off single sensory (sympathetic) fibers that extend into the epithelium. As in other squamous epithelia (*e.g.* skin), these follow a zigzag course as they pass through the epithelium toward the luminal surface. Anatomically, these appear to be placed so as to respond to stimuli at that surface.

1.3.2.5. Extramural Nerves

The two vagus nerves pass from the skull through the neck and into the thorax alongside the esophagus. They extend down to a point about one-third of the length of that organ below the pharyngoesophageal junction where they break up into a few large branches that soon fuse again and then branch and fuse repeatedly, forming a plexus of coarse fiber bundles that surrounds the organ to a level just above the diaphragm (Fig. **11**). At this point, the bundles fuse again to form two to four nerve trunks, the vagal trunks that pass into the abdomen through the esophageal hiatus in the diaphragm, adjacent to the esophagogastric sphincter.

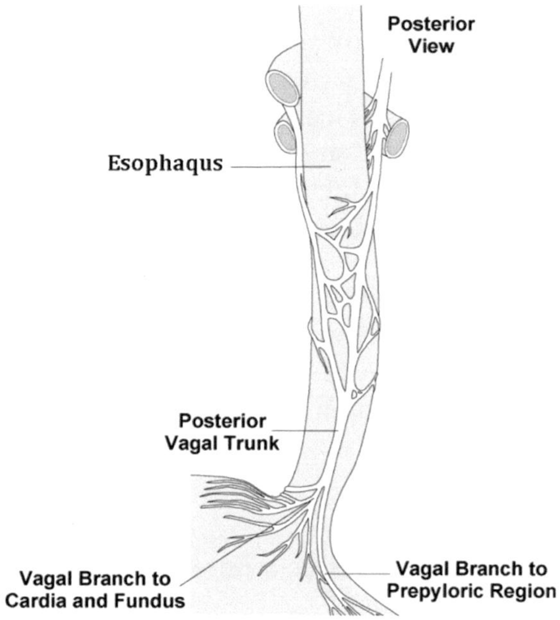

Figure 11: A sketch of the vagus nerves, the esophageal plexus, and the vagal trunks (shown from the posterior).

The network of vagal bundles surrounding the esophagus, the esophageal plexus, mingles nerve fibers from the right and left vagus nerves. It gives off small nerve fiber bundles that enter directly into the muscular wall of the organ. Some of these nerve fibers end in the myenteric plexus. Others pass through the myenteric plexus, to enter the stomach within the wall of the gut, supplying the myenteric plexus of the rostral parts of that organ (Fig. **12**).

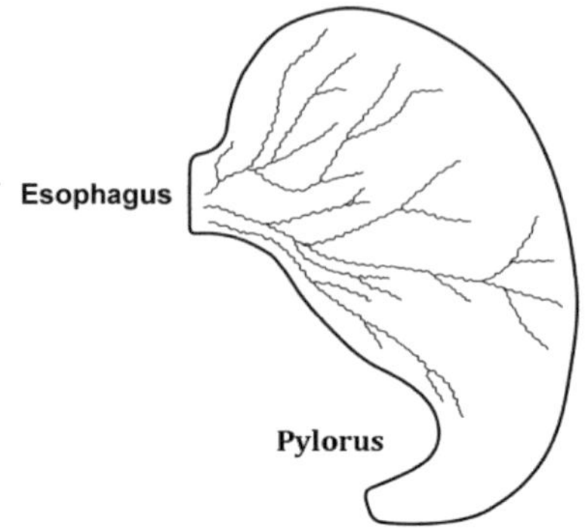

Figure 12: A sketch of the vagal nerve branches that pass from the esophagus into the rostral part of the stomach.

1.3.3. Stomach and Pyloric Sphincter

In embryogenesis, the gut first appears as a collapsible cylindrical tube of uniform caliber. The stomach arises very early in embryogenesis, beginning as a widening at the rostral end of this basic form. This enlargement occurs on the left side. With embryonic development, this dilatation grows to become a saccule, the fundus of the stomach, and the primordial tube elongates and rotates to produce the transversely oriented asymmetric oblate spheroid of the mature animal.

The initial rostral dilation becomes the gastric fundus. It allows for the storage of ingested materials, ending the necessity for the organism to take in nutrients continuously. The caudal part of the embryonic dilatation retains a cylindrical and conical form as the embryo grows. It becomes the antrum of the stomach. It functions to grind and mix the luminal contents.

1.3.3.1. Musculature

The rostral part of the stomach possesses a third muscle layer, called the oblique muscle layer (Fig. **13**).

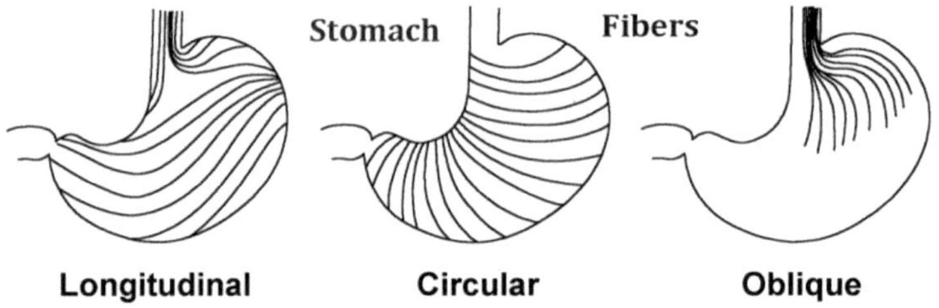

Figure 13: A diagram of the three layers of muscle in the stomach.

This arrangement reflects the storage function of this region. The oblique muscle layer lies on the luminal (inner) side of the circular layer of muscle. A thin sheet of connective tissue separates the oblique and circular muscle layers throughout the fundus but they fuse in the part of the organ that separates the fundus from the antrum. Thus, the oblique muscle layer seems to originate from the inner circular muscle layer, arising as a laminar splitting, with its fibers looping in such a way as to enclose the saccular part of the stomach, the fundus. When its cells shorten in contraction, this oblique muscle layer diminishes the volume of the fundus by reducing its radii quasi-symmetrically, pulling the apex of the fundus toward the antrum.

The circular muscle layer of the stomach thickens progressively toward its junction with the duodenum. An even greater thickening characterizes the most distal segment, a region generally called the pylorus or the pyloric sphincter. This muscular structure is not simply a ring of thickened muscle encircling the lumen. Rather, it is one loop (the smaller loop) of an asymmetrical double torus, a geometrical configuration resembling a bent figure-of-eight, the other larger loop of which encircles the antrum obliquely some distance above the gastroduodenal junction (Fig. **14**).

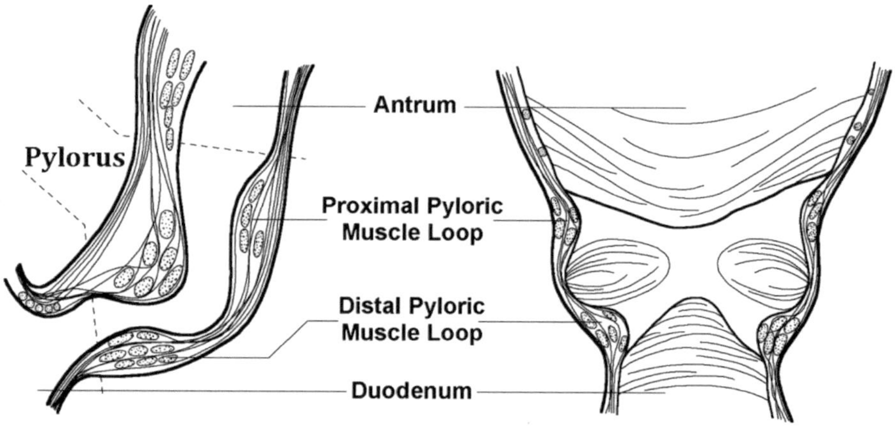

Figure 14: A diagram of the double torus of muscle in the pylorus and gastric antrum.

The two loops of this double torus are joined along the right side of the antrum, on the side generally called the "lesser curvature". Thus, contraction of this torus must both narrow the lumen at the pyloric opening and also narrow and angulate the organ between the distal antrum and the rostral part of the antrum. This probably explains, in part, the observation that the stomach may vary in configuration from a "cow's-horn" shape to a "J " shape.

The outer longitudinal muscle layer of the stomach possesses a special relationship to the pylorus. Most of this muscle layer inserts into the thickened muscle of the pyloric loop of the circular muscle layer. However, a very small part of the longitudinal musculature, the outermost layer of cells, passes over the outside of the pyloric loop to join with the longitudinal muscle layer of the duodenum. This arrangement implies that the longitudinal muscle layer of the stomach shortens the antrum as it contracts.

The interstitial cells of Cajal are distributed throughout the thickness of the muscle in the gastric circular layer. They are very much more abundant in the antrum than in the fundus. They exhibit a gradient in density, there being essentially none in the circular musculature next to the esophagogastric junction, a maximal density in the region of the pylorus, and intermediate densities of distribution at intermediate levels throughout the stomach.

1.3.3.2. Connective Tissue

The stomach hangs in a mesentery, a fold of the peritoneum encasing the organ and attaching it to the posterior wall of the abdomen. The core of this fold, a shelf of connective tissue containing nerves and blood vessels, is covered on both sides by the serosa. The presence of a mesentery frees the organ of encumbrances in its movements. The phrenoesophageal ligament (see above) fixes the stomach loosely to the diaphragm at its rostral end, and the retroperitoneal position of the duodenum ties the caudal end of the stomach to the posterior abdominal wall.

The thin sheet of connective tissue that separates the oblique and circular muscle layers in the gastric fundus contains no plexus of nerves. The plane between the longitudinal and circular muscle layers conforms to the general description given above in the section on the general structure of the gut.

The very thick submucosa of the stomach allows the substantial mucosa in the rostral parts of the organ to be thrown into broad folds (often called the gastric rugae) that extend in the axial direction when the organ is only partly filled. Filling of the organ effaces these rugae. The submucosa and mucosa of the antrum are thinner and less generous so no rugae occur there.

1.3.3.3. Intramural Nerves

The myenteric plexus is very sparse in the gastric fundus as compared to the antrum, but the antrum contains the densest distribution of myenteric plexus neurons to be found anywhere in the alimentary canal. In both regions, the plexus forms the classical polygonal network of ganglia and interganglionic fascicles.

The intramural extensions of the vagal nerves that pass from the esophagus into the stomach extend and ramify around the fundus. This pattern minimizes their vulnerability to the possibility of breakage with the radial expansion of the fundus that occurs in gastric filling.

Despite the massive secretion that characterizes the gastric mucosa, the submucosal plexus is sparse in the stomach as compared to the small intestine. This fact suggests that the myenteric plexus and the extrinsic innervation may be more important in the control of secretion by the gastric epithelium.

1.3.3.4. Epithelium

The gastric mucosa is thick and succulent as compared to that in other parts of the gut. The gastric epithelium is dedicated to the secretion of a large volume of fluid, gastric acid as well as mucus, and this requires epithelial glands that enlarge the whole mucosa, thickening both the epithelium and the lamina propria. They even thicken the submucosa into which the epithelial glands protrude. The combined mass of the mucosa and submucosa contributes to the formation of the thick folds, the gastric rugae that are so characteristic a feature of the stomach upon gross inspection. The mass of the combined mucosa-submucosa is much diminished in the caudal part of the stomach, the antrum, in part because the secretory function of the epithelium is so much greater in the more rostral regions of the organ.

1.3.3.5. Extramural Nerves

The craniosacral innervation of the stomach is entirely vagal. In contrast to the vagal innervation of the gastric fundus, which comes especially through vagal extensions by way of the esophagus, the vagal innervation of the antrum enters the organ from the outside, from vagal branches that depart from the vagal trunks well below the diaphragm on the right side.

The thoracolumbar innervation arises principally from the celiac ganglion (the most rostral element in the complex of prevertebral or retroperitoneal ganglia) passing to the stomach through the perivascular nerve plexus that follows the branches of the celiac artery. A small component also passes to the stomach through the vagus nerves, these thoracolumbar fibers entering into the vagus nerves in the neck.

1.3.4. Small Intestine and Ileocecal Sphincter

The general scheme of the structure of the gastrointestinal tract essentially describes the whole of the small intestine. The organ is, however, not quite uniform throughout its length in that it appears to be a little narrower, in general, at its caudal extremity than it is more rostrally.

1.3.4.1. Muscle

There is a slight gradient in the thickness of the main muscle coats exists so that the muscle layers appear to be a little thicker at the rostral end than at the caudal end.

In the small intestine, the interstitial cells of Cajal lie especially concentrated in a single plane within the substance of the circular muscle layer. They appear to be a little more numerous in the duodenum than they are in the ileum.

1.3.4.2. Connective Tissue

The duodenum is relatively fixed in position, being retroperitoneal while the rest of the small intestine, like the stomach, is suspended from the posterior abdominal wall by a mesentery. This tethers the small intestine so that its freedom of movement is somewhat restricted.

This intestinal mesentery, like all the mesenteries of the abdomen, consists of a shelf of connective tissue, covered on both sides by the serosa and holding the vessels and extrinsic nerves that must pass from the posterior abdominal wall to the gut. At the most rostral level of this small intestinal mesentery, it forms a special band, the ligament of Treitz that ties the small intestine to the posterior abdominal wall and holds the spleen and the splenic flexure of the large intestine in place. At the most caudal limit of the intestine, the ileocecal junction, the shortness of the intestinal mesenteric attachment ties that end of the small intestine in position.

Between the ligament of Treitz and the ileocolic junction, the breadth of the mesentery allows considerable movement of the small intestine within the abdomen. The mesenteric attachment of the small intestine to the posterior abdominal wall does not affect the freedom of movement of the organ as its musculature contracts. However, the mesentery keeps the long and pliable intestine oriented in such a way as to prevent gross deformations. Too much mobility would allow this extremely motile tube to form obstructive twists or knots, while the considerable packing of the long tube into the small space of the abdomen requires some capacity for loops to move about.

1.3.4.3. Epithelium

The epithelium of the small intestine forms finger-like or leaf-like protrusions, the intestinal villi that greatly increase the surface available for absorption. These villi are actually formed by the lamina propria over which the epithelium lies as a single layer of cells. The villi give the mucosa a certain thickness that makes for the formation of thick folds in the collapsed organ.

The mucosa itself is formed into fixed semi-circular folds, the *plicae.* These represent structures of the submucosa over which the mucosa lies.

The actual absorptive cells of the small intestine cover the villi as a single layer. Since the villi are closely packed, the circulation of fluid over the absorptive surface at the sides of the villi would be compromised were it not for micro-movements known to occur in the villi. Only the general nature of such movements is known. They pump up and down individually and independently in a motion that must enhance this circulation. They also shift *en masse* in waves. Such mucosal movements, imparted by the contractions of the mucosal muscle, must exchange the fluid mass at the absorptive surface, thereby reducing the unstirred layer at this surface. Since the diffusion of molecules in this layer is the rate-limiting step in intestinal absorption, this stirring must be critical in nutrition.

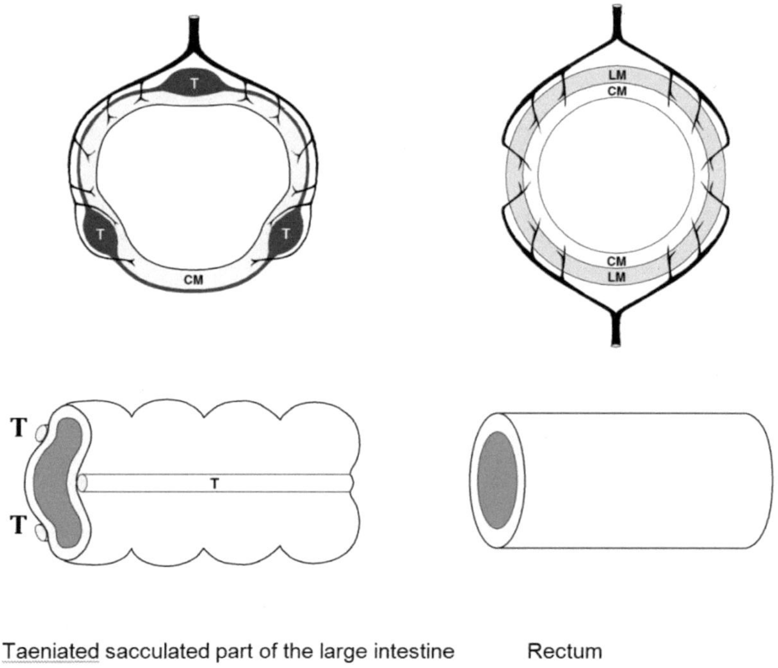

Figure 15: The musculature of the large intestine as shown in cross section. In man, most of the organ possesses three thickened bundles of longitudinally oriented muscle, the taeniae, as diagrammed on the left. In the most caudal part of the human large intestine, the rectum, the three taeniae spread and fuse so that the longitudinal muscle layer is uniformly thick about the organ.

1.3.5. Large Intestine and Anal Sphincter

1.3.5.1. Musculature

The outer or longitudinal muscle layer forms three thick bundles, the taeniae of the large intestine that extend from the tip of the cecum to the rostral end of the rectum (Fig. **15**). A very thin layer of the longitudinal muscular layer covers the surface of the large intestine between these taeniae.

The circular muscle layer forms narrow thickenings, the haustral markings, at fairly regular intervals along the colon. The wall of the organ bulges between these haustral markings as well as between the three taeniae. The colon, which is the whole of the large intestine, except for the cecum and rectum, is consequently sacculated in appearance, the saccules being defined both by the haustral markings and by the restriction that the taeniae impose (Fig. **16**).

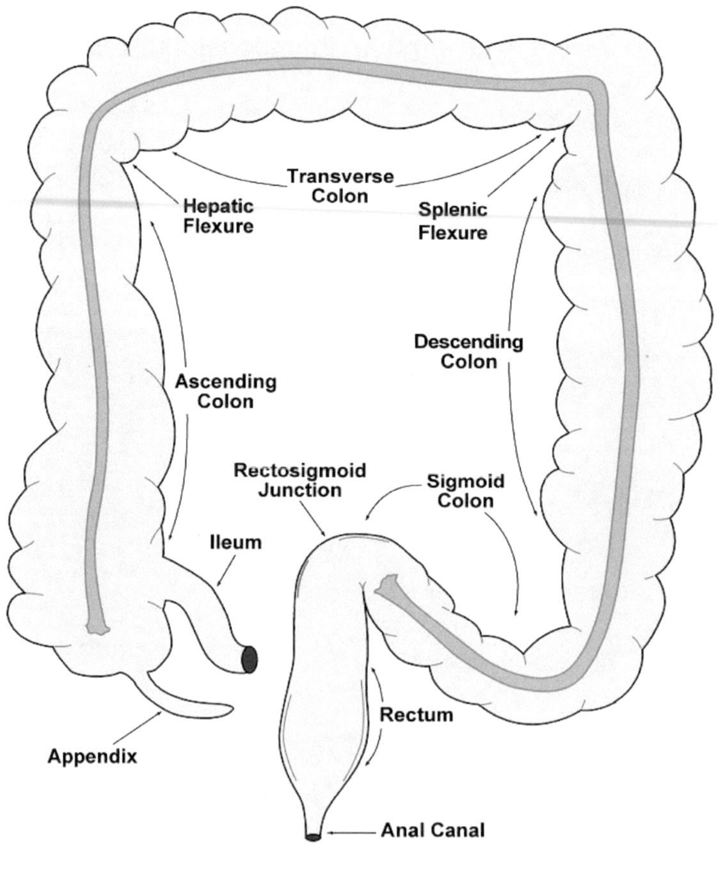

Figure 16: The gross appearance of the human large intestine.

The circular muscle layer thickens at the caudal limit of the large intestine to form the internal anal sphincter. This sphincter lies enclosed within but separate from the external anal sphincter, a torus of muscle that is a part of the pelvic floor.

As a somatic muscular structure derived from somatic muscle of the pelvic floor, the external anal sphincter is not actually a part of the gastrointestinal tract. The nature, position, and function of the external anal sphincter give it the responsibility for voluntary continence.

1.3.5.2. Connective Tissue

The large intestine is fixed in position at several points, but this fixation seems not to impede the movements that result from the contractions of its intrinsic musculature. However, the points of fixation keep the whole organ loosely in place. The mesentery is particularly short at the ileocecal junction, at the hepatic flexure, and at the splenic flexure where it forms structures sometimes called ligaments. These points establish the angulations called the flexures of the large intestine. The colonic mesentery is a little broader along the ascending and descending colon and even more generous along the transverse colon. At the rectosigmoid junction, the organ becomes extraperitoneal so that the most caudal part of the organ, the rectum, lies packed with the other pelvic viscera within the confines of the lesser pelvis and surrounded by a connective tissue matrix.

1.3.5.3. Epithelium

The epithelium of the large intestine is dedicated mainly to the absorption of water and the production of mucus. The volumes involved are generally less than those of absorption and secretion in the more rostral organs. Accordingly, the epithelium is not so thick in this organ as it is in the stomach and small intestine. When the organ is collapsed, the mucosa tends to form thinner folds than do the other organs.

1.3.5.4. Extrinsic Innervation

The craniosacral innervation of the large intestine arises from the pelvic plexus, a network of nerves formed by the branching of the pelvic nerves. The colonic branches from this plexus pierce the colonic wall at the level of the rectosigmoid junction and branch there to form a series of large trunks that extend in the rostral direction within the plane of the myenteric plexus up to the midpoint of the organ (Fig. **17**).

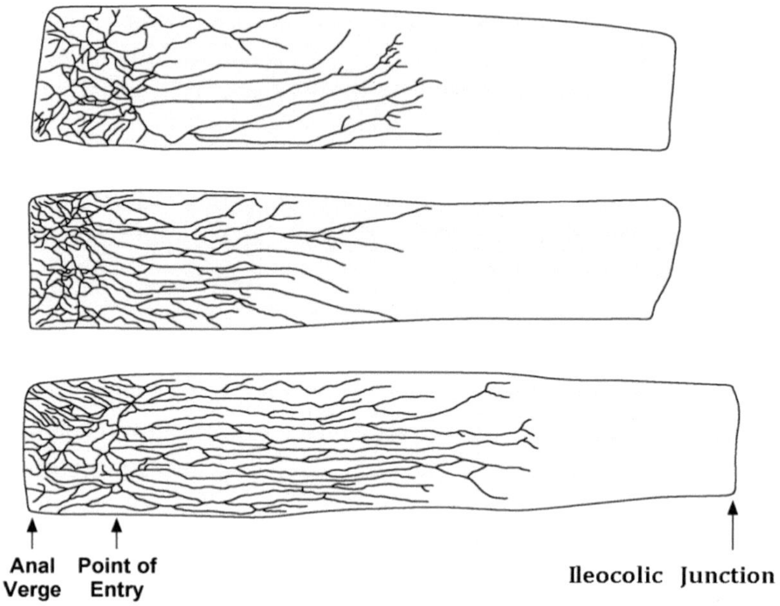

Figure 17: A diagram of the distribution of the extrinsic innervation of the large intestine. The anal verge, at the left, is the level where the rectal epithelium abuts the skin. These are tracings from three cat intestines showing how the extrinsic (parasympathetic) nerves, after having pierced through the longitudinal muscle layer at the colorectal junction, extend between the two principal muscle layers. They distribute nerve fibers to the ganglia of the myenteric plexus of the large intestine from the anal verge to the midpoint of the colon.

They supply nerve fibers to the ganglia of the myenteric plexus. Some branches extend toward the anus, forming a plexus of nerves of extrinsic origin within the intermuscular plane throughout the rectum, where there are comparatively few intrinsic nerves.

1.3.6. The Biliary Tract

The general function of the biliary tract is the transfer of fluids from the pancreas, liver, and gallbladder to the duodenum.

In embryogenesis, the biliary tract develops as a bud sprouting from the simple tube that constitutes the primitive gastrointestinal tract. It remains, in essence, a blind tunnel although it evolves into an extensively branched tree with highly specialized structures at the extremities of its blind branches. These are the pancreas, liver, and gallbladder that serve critical secretory and excretory functions. The tract also develops specialization in parts of the conduit itself that serve specific mechanical functions. The spiral valve of Heister, a convolution in the duct system from the gallbladder to the bile duct appears to have a mechanical function, perhaps to enhance the resistance to outflow from the gallbladder.

1.3.6.1. Musculature

The system of ducts that form the biliary tract, the bile duct and its branches, lack an intrinsic musculature except for the thick and short segment adjacent to the duodenum. Here, a circular muscle layer, the sphincter of Oddi, makes up a single functional entity surrounding both the pancreatic and bile ducts. Elsewhere, most of the wall of the biliary tract consists of a rather tough layer of connective tissue forming comparatively rigid passive conduits. The wall of the gallbladder, however, contains poorly organized muscle bundles within a loose connective tissue stroma.

1.3.6.2. Connective Tissue and Epithelium

Throughout the biliary tract, there is a submucosa of loose connective tissue over which the epithelium lies. The epithelium is cuboidal, a term that denotes the shape of the individual epithelial cells. This shape allows them to flatten, in accordance with the large changes in intraluminal volume possible in the system.

1.3.6.3. Intramural Nerves

There is no intramural innervation in the biliary tract. Instead, the intrinsic innervation simply lies outside the system of ducts as an extension of the intestinal myenteric plexus.

REFERENCES

Most of the information covered in this chapter can be explored further by the consultation of standard textbooks of anatomy and histology. The following references contain observations of high relevance for this chapter.

[1] Christensen J, Wingate DL. A Guide to Gastrointestinal Motilty. Bristol, London, Boston: Wright PSG 1983.

[2] Christensen J, Rick GA. Nerve Cell Density in Submucous, Plexus throughout the Gut of Cat and Opossum. Gastroenterology 1985; 89: 1064-1069.

[3] Christensen J, Rick GA. The Distribution of Myelinated, Nerves in the Ascending Nerves and Myenteric. Plexus of the Cat Colon. Am J Anat 1987; 178: 250-258.

[4] Christensen J, Rick G.A, Lowe L.S. Distributions of Interstitial Cells of Cajal in Stomach and Colon of Cat, Dog, Ferret, Opossum, Rat, Guinea Pig and Rabbit. J Auton. Nerv Syst 1992; 37: 47-56.

[5] Christensen J, Rick GA, Soll DJ. Intramural Nerves and Interstitial Cells Revealed by the Champy-Maillet Stain in the Opossum Esophagus. J Auton. Nerv Syst 1987; 14: 137-151.

[6] Christensen J, Rick GA, Robison BA, Stiles M.J, Wix MA. The Arrangement of the Myenteric Plexus throughout the Gastrointestinal Tract of the Opossum. Gastroenterology 1983; 85: 890-899.

[7] Christensen J. Origin of Sensation in the Esophagus. Am J Physiol (Gastrointestinal and Liver Physiology) 1984; 9: G221-G225.

[8] Christensen J. The Forms of Argyrophilic Ganglion Cells in the Myenteric Plexus throughout the Gastrointestinal Tract of the Opossum. J Auton Nerv Syst 1988; 24: 251-260.

[9] Furness JB, Costa M. The Enteric Nervous System. Edinburgh, London, Melbourne, New York: Churchill Livingstone 1987.

[10] Gabella G. Structure of the Autonomic Nervous System. New York; Chapman and Hall. London, The Halsted Press, John Wiley & Sons 1976.

[11] Kumar D, Wingate DL. An Illustrated Guide to Gastrointestinal Motility. Edinburgh, London, Madrid, Melbourne, New York and Tokyo; Churchill, Livingstone 2nd Edition 1993.

[12] Phillips SF, Pemberton JH, Shorter RG. The Large Intestine. Physiology, Pathophysiology, Disease, New York: Raven Press 1991.

[13] Stevens CE. Comparative Physiology of the Vertebrate Digestive System. Cambridge, New York, New Rochelle, Melbourne, Sydney: Cambridge University Press 1988.

CHAPTER 2

Biomechanical Theory

Abstract: This chapter aims to give the reader a basic understanding of mechanical theory, especially related to stresses and strains and how these parameters should be interpreted in comparison with more commonly used distensibility measures. The bioengineering way of thinking is introduced and references are made to functional aspects of the gastrointestinal tract. In order to understand the biomechanical complexity it is important to know about the complex anatomical features of the gastrointestinal tract as outlined in chapter 1 of this book.

Keywords: Bioengineering, biomechanics, distensibility, esophagus, fluid flow, force, intestine, residual strain, stomach, strain, stress, zero-stress state.

2.1. THE MEANING OF BIOMECHANICS

Mechanics, the study of the motion of matter and the forces that cause such motion, has been applied to the analysis of dynamic systems from atoms to solar systems. The analysis of deformation, stress, and stability of thin-walled tubes, a classical physics and engineering subject, occupied such pioneers as Bernoulli, Cauchy, Euler, Flügge, Kirchhoff, Reissner, and Timeshenko.

Many descriptions separate the study of solid mechanics from fluid mechanics. In general a discrete, finite, and time-independent deformation is elicited when a constant force is transmitted to a solid material. In a fluid the same force causes a time-dependent and continuous response called flow. Hence, a fluid is a material that is unable to withstand a static shear stress. A fluid responds with an irrecoverable flow, unlike an elastic solid, which responds to a shear stress with a recoverable deformation. The fluid-solid state is characterized by an intermediate response constituting viscoelastic material behavior. Analysis of the basic relations between stress and strain is fundamental in solid mechanics. In fluid mechanics, the variables needed to define a fluid and its environment are pressure, density, viscosity, velocity, body force and time. Fluids include gases and liquids. Liquids are typically considered to be incompressible whereas gases are considered to be compressible. Fluid flow can be either turbulent or laminar.

Biomechanics, being based on engineering and physics principles, requires understanding of biology in addition to mechanics, mathematics, and statistics. The purpose of biomechanics is to explain the mechanical behavior of living organisms. When applied to gastrointestinal biology, it requires a thorough

Hans Gregersen and James Christensen

understanding of anatomy, structure, function, pathophysiology and symptoms. Gastrointestinal tract complexity demands a multidisciplinary approach using experimental, analytical and numerical methods.

The gastrointestinal tract can be viewed as a complex mechanical device but the scientific study of its mechanics is yet immature. Medicine and physiology have until now disregarded gut mechanics as a matter for serious consideration, despite the high prevalence of disordered mechanics in clinical gastroenterology. Perhaps this only reflects the neglect of physics, mechanical engineering and mathematics in the fundamental education of biologists. Gastrointestinal motor function disorders to some degree characterize many if not most patients with complaints from digestive system. For example almost all diseases of the esophagus exhibit some kind of abnormality in mechanical function in that organ. Furthermore, mechanical dysfunction often complicates the connective tissue diseases, diabetes and neurological disorders.

The basic relation between stress and strain is an important concept in biomechanics. Many artificial (engineered) materials are characterized by simple stress-strain relations due to homogeneous material that behaves in an isotropic manner and with infinitesimal deformation even at large stresses. Many engineering materials behave this way, and obey Hooke's law with Young's modulus as the proportionality constant between stress and strain. However, biological tissues including the gastrointestinal wall differ in most ways from the common engineered materials that exhibit such behavior. The gastrointestinal wall specifically exhibits or possesses

- complex geometry
- multi-layered structure
- heterogeneous materials
- viscoelastic behavior, *i.e.* the tissue has the mechanical properties of both fluids and solids
- anisotropic behavior (mechanical behavior that differs in one direction or dimension from another)
- non-linear stress-strain curves at large deformations
- intrinsic active properties of muscle tissue and the associated nerves

The difficulty increases with consideration of the fact that the gastrointestinal tract is a series of organs exhibiting somewhat different behaviors. For example, the mechanical characteristics of the wall of the stomach clearly differ from those of the esophagus wall. Differences exist even between one region of a single organ and another region, such as between the gastric antrum and fundus.

The mechanical analysis of the gut wall is much more difficult than that of structures made of the usual engineering materials due to this complexity. In fact the composition of the gastrointestinal tract is so complex that simple and rudimentary measures as compliance (the pressure-volume curve slope) are used to describe its mechanical properties. However, a compliance measure is insufficient in a mechanical analysis. It can easily lead to erroneous conclusions about the material behavior. A stress-strain analysis for any material requires simplifying assumptions to reduce the number of experiments and the complexity of the analysis. Such assumptions, however, cannot be chosen randomly. They must relate to the scientific problem, and the validity should be tested during the process.

The history of gastrointestinal biomechanics can be traced to the seventeenth century when Borelli first thought to consider the gastrointestinal tract as a biomechanical system. However, not until the late nineteenth century was the mechanical function of the gastrointestinal tract studied seriously by biologists. Nothnagel in 1882 [1] and Mall in 1896 [2] demonstrated the peristaltic reflex long before Bayliss and Starling, who get the credit for its first description, called "the law of the intestine" in 1899-1901 [3, 4]. Only after that did the technique for the study of gut muscle *in vitro* develop enough to allow the examination of its active and passive mechanical behavior and to permit its application in pharmacology, where the technique remains in use. Walter B. Cannon's book, "The Mechanical Factors of Digestion" from 1911 [5], was a milestone, and Trendelenburg's model in 1917 for studying peristalsis [6] was an important development. After that, however, gastroenterology was sidestepped by the advances that took place in the mechanical study of other tissues, especially in orthopedics and cardiovascular physiology.

Mechanical studies of gastrointestinal properties and function have suffered from inaccessibility of the gut, requiring development of specialized methods for examination *in vivo*. Recently, bag distension techniques for biomechanical analysis, such as the impedance planimetric method for studies *in vivo*, are becoming established in physiological studies of the gastrointestinal tract.

Developing methods, using non-invasive imaging with MR-scanning, ultrasound, and multi-slice CT-scanning in combination with bag distension, are emerging for future application.

Only a few research groups have treated the gastrointestinal tract from a modern bioengineering viewpoint. Publications have come from Fung, Tozeren, Srivastava and Srivastava, and Metry [7-10], among others. Macagno and Christensen worked on duodenal contractility and flow from 1970 to about 1985, some of the work published in journals while the rest remains in the theses of students [11]. Brasseur has written extensively on flow and contractility in the esophagus and stomach over the past two decades and provided valuable mechanical models of the esophagogastric junction [12-14]. Miftakhov examined gastrointestinal peristalsis and its regulation, and other behaviors, with the use of bioengineering principles [15]. Gregersen and coworkers have focused on the development of new biomechanical equipment and methods, on the residual stresses and strains in the gastrointestinal tract, on the *in vivo* length-tension characteristics of gastrointestinal muscle, bilayer models and mechanosensation [16-21]. For understanding biomechanical aspects and assumption in biomechanical analysis it is, in addition to the literature referenced above, also worthwhile to consult literature by Do Carmo [22] and Regen [23] and the books by Fung of biomechanics and continuum mechanics [7, 24].

2.1.1. Application of Gastrointestinal Biomechanics

As a mechanical system, the gastrointestinal tract serves primarily mechanical functions. In this to some degree self-regulated system, distension of the tract can elicit both excitation and inhibition of muscle contraction by way of extrinsic and intrinsic reflex circuits, as well as sensations like pain through central nervous connections of the digestive tract. Afferent neurons activated by mechano-sensitive receptors in the digestive tract wall are the sensing elements. From a mechanical point of view these receptors are yet not well characterized.

Bioengineering and biomechanical principles are applicable to almost any problem related to gastrointestinal function and motor dysfunction. Mechanical analysis of the operation of the gastrointestinal tract will be important to advance the understanding of wide-ranging set of matters such as

- the elastic and viscoelastic (passive) properties of the wall
- the wall responses to mechanoreceptor stimulation

- the peristaltic reflexes
- the mechanics of bolus transport
- the origin of gastrointestinal perceptions or sensations
- the nature and origin of tone in smooth muscle
- the development and growth of the gut
- remodeling of the geometry and biomechanical properties in the gut
- the origin of mechanical dysfunction related gastrointestinal diseases
- new clinical test development for mechanical dysfunction in the gut

These matters are interrelated, as will be evident from a reading of later chapters. A bioengineering approach to gastrointestinal mechanics should allow a better definition of the relationships between mechanical stimulation, the neuronal activity that regulates motor functions, the muscular activity that expresses neuronal activity, and the flows of the fluid contents of the tract that result from the wall movements generated by the muscle.

2.2. THE BIOENGINEERING APPROACH

Bioengineering principles have begun to enter the minds of physiologists only in recent decades. This has happened relatively fast in cardiovascular and musculoskeletal physiology but not in gastroenterology. Bioengineering, the application of engineering knowledge and methods to biology and medicine, has developed as a discipline because of the recognition that organisms as they carry out a wide range of physiological and mechanical functions must contend with the physical characteristics of their environment. Most work in bioengineering has been done by electrical engineers in the development of electronic instruments for clinical medicine. Bioengineering has proved valuable in rehabilitation medicine, in gait analysis and in the development of artificial limbs, as well as in the cardiovascular field.

Biomechanics is necessary in bioengineering for the study of biological systems that have mechanical functions. Biomechanics relates not only to such obvious matters as gait analysis, somatic muscle function and cardiovascular function but also to the visceral organs with the fluids that move in the gastrointestinal and genitourinary tracts.

The term gastrointestinal motility is defined as the characteristic ability of the gastrointestinal tract to generate motions. It encompasses a wide array of subjects including wall movements, the factors that control the motions, and the movements of the luminal contents induced by the motions. Consequently, biomechanics is key in studying gastrointestinal motility, being necessary both for describing how the intent of the neural control system is expressed and how flow of the gastrointestinal contents is produced.

Any measurement of forces or motions of the gastrointestinal wall must be treated as a biomechanical measurement, requiring a rigorous mechanical analysis based on bioengineering principles. The last decade has seen an increased tendency for students of gastrointestinal motility to gather data on the distensibility of gastrointestinal organs. This popularity stems largely from the ease with which the data are gathered. If they are to be interpreted correctly, the data must be treated according to the basic principles of biomechanics.

2.2.1. Eight Steps in the Development of a Biomechanical Model

In this book we emphasize a rational approach adopted and modified from physics and engineering by Fung for the study of problems in biomechanics [7]. Important problems in gastrointestinal physiology and pathophysiology call for the most careful considerations of the geometry, structure, biological factors and mechanical properties of the gut and their application in constitutive equations, in the manner familiar to bioengineers. Boundary-value problems can be formulated and solved, further testing can be done and the data compared to theory. The developed theory can be used to predict tissue behavior in disease and in response to medical and surgical intervention. The biomechanical approach to the study of the gastrointestinal structure and function represents a potentially important multidisciplinary approach that adds new insights to our understanding of gastrointestinal structural design and function. The bioengineering approach advocated by Fung can be formulated as eight steps:

1. The geometric configuration must be studied first. This includes the morphology of the organism; the anatomy of the organ; and the structure and composition of the tissue.

2. The biophysical properties of the materials and tissues that are involved must be determined. Problems in isolating the tissue for testing or keeping the organ alive during the experiment may make this step difficult. Moreover, the mechanical behavior of biological tissues is complex with large deformation and nonlinear properties.

3. The governing differential of integral equations must be derived on the basis of the fundamental laws of physics (conservation of mass, momentum, and energy, and Maxwell's equations) and the constitutive equations of the materials.

4. The environment in which an organ functions must be understood in order to set realistic boundary conditions.

5. With the approach mentioned above, the boundary-value problems (differential equations with appropriate initial and boundary conditions) can be solved by experiments, analytically or numerically.

6. Physiological experiments to test the solutions of the boundary-value problems must be performed. The mathematical problem must be reformulated and resolved, if necessary, to assure that the theory and experiment correspond.

7. The experimental results must be compared with the corresponding theoretical results. If the hypotheses made in the theory are justified, the numerical values of the undetermined coefficients in the constitutive equations can be determined.

8. The outcome of other boundary-value problems associated with the same basic equations can then be predicted using the validated theory. With this basic information, biomechanics can be used for invention of new devices and methods for intervention.

A closer look at this plan and these eight points in the light of what we now think about gastrointestinal motor function reveals how little we actually know. The relevant anatomy and structure of the gastrointestinal are quite well known but the data have generally been collected empirically rather than with the above approach in mind. Only now are data appearing on the mechanical properties of the gastrointestinal tract, but it is still often acquired empirically.

What needs to be done in respect to the study of gastrointestinal mechanics is quite straightforward. The constitutive equations, *i.e.* the 3D stress-strain relationships of the gastrointestinal tissues, must be determined. With the constitutive equations, the physical stresses and strains distributions in the organs *in vivo*, and the function of fluid movement and bolus transport in the gastrointestinal tract can be analyzed by continuum mechanics methods. The analytical results will relate the stress and function of the gastrointestinal tract with the geometric parameters of the structure. Determining the constitutive equations is not as difficult as it may seem because the mathematical forms of many soft tissues are known. If the idea can be confirmed that the constitutive equations of gastrointestinal tissues are like those of other soft tissues, then identifying the mathematical constants of the gastrointestinal tissues only remains. Determinations of the geometry and the solid mechanical properties of the gastrointestinal tissues are, however, only the first steps in the direction of a full understanding of the nature of flow in the gastrointestinal tract.

2.3. SOLID MECHANICS

2.3.1. Definitions of Terms

Determination of the stresses and strains in biological materials when forces are acting on them is one principal objective in tissue biomechanics. A complete picture of the biomechanical behavior is obtained by determination of these quantities over a range of loads, from a stage approximating the unloaded state up to loads causing failure. A study of the force-deformation relationship is demanded by the fact that forces applied to solids deform them. The gastrointestinal tract as well as other biological tissues express mechanical properties between solid and fluid properties *i.e.* anisotropy prevails due to the heterogeneous laminated structure of the gut wall, the deformation is finite, the stress-strain relation is non-linear, and time-dependent (viscoelastic) behavior is evident. Due to the high water content, these biological tissues express mechanical properties of both viscous fluid and an elastic solid. The biomechanical properties are time-dependent since the stress-strain response does not occur instantly. The corresponding stresses induced in the wall decrease with time when the material is suddenly strained and the strain is kept constant. This phenomenon is named stress relaxation. Likewise the material continues to deform if the material is suddenly stressed and the stress is maintained constant. This phenomenon is named creep. Furthermore, if the tissue is subjected to a cyclic loading, the stress-strain relationship in the loading process is different from that in the unloading process. This phenomenon is called hysteresis. Stress relaxation, creep, and hysteresis are all viscoelastic features, as described in more detail later in this chapter.

The scientist must consider the structure and geometry of the tissues when dealing with the mechanical properties of the gastrointestinal tract. These aspects of the system are dealt with in Chapter 1. This chapter serves to provide the basic theory for treating the gastrointestinal tissue from a mechanical point of view. Such a theory is necessary to understand the passive properties of the gastrointestinal wall, to understand the gastrointestinal tract as a passive conduit. The passive properties must be understood before the active properties, the muscle contractions and the flows they produce, can be considered. Most of the terms used in this chapter and in the next chapters are defined in Table **1**.

Table 1. Some common terms used in solid and fluid mechanics

Compliance	The ratio between pressure change and volume change.
Composite materials	A composite material consists of two of more phases on a macroscopic scale. Many types of composites exist, for example fibers embedded in a matrix or laminated structures.
Constitutive equation	A mechanical constitutive equation describes the mechanical properties of a material, also known as the stress-strain relation.
Deformation	Forces applied to solids cause deformation (strain). For elastic deformation, the material returns to its initial state when the stress is removed. The deformation is plastic if the material does not return to the initial state.
Density	The mass of fluid per unit volume.
Elastic modulus	The constant of proportionality between stress and strain. For a homogenous linearly elastic material Hooke's law applies.
Force	A force has both magnitude and direction making it a vector quantity. It is measured in the SI units of newton. A force is any interaction tending to change the motion of an object. Hence, a force can cause an object with mass to change its velocity, *i.e.* to accelerate. Force can also be described by intuitive concepts such as a push or a pull.
Incompressible	An incompressible fluid is characterized by constant density.
Isotropy	An isotropic material has properties which are the same in all directions or are independent of the orientation of the reference axis. In anisotropic materials the mechanical properties depend on directions. Many biological tissues are anisotropic because of their heterogeneous, layered structure.
Laminar	An organized flow field that can be described with streamlines. The viscous stresses must dominate over the fluid inertia stresses in order for laminar flow to be permissible.
Membrane tension	membrane tension is the uniform stress multiplied with wall thickness, expressed as force per unit length. Instead of membrane tension, some scientists use "stress resultants" or "membrane stress resultants" to recognize the fact that they are the stress integrals throughout the membrane wall thickness.
Newtonian fluid	A viscous fluid whose shear stresses are a linear function of the fluid strain rate. Most fluids do not behave as Newtonian fluids.
Preconditioning	Loading and unloading are repeated for a number of cycles In mechanical testing of living tissues *in vitro* until the stress-strain relation becomes stabilized and repeatable results are obtained.
Pressure	A measure of the force per unit area exerted. The SI unit is N m^{-2} or pascal.

Table 1: contd…

Residual strain	The strain at the no-load state (where absent external forces) with reference to the stress-free (zero-stress) state.
Strain	Forces applied to solids result in deformation or strain. Strain is a tensor quantity. Consider uni-axial conditions such as a string with initial length L_0 and stretched length L. It is useful to describe the change by dimensionless ratios such as L/L_0 or $(L-L_0)/L_0$ since it eliminates the absolute length from consideration. Elongation causes tensile (positive) strain while shortening causes compressive (negative) strain.
Stress	The force per unit surface area that the part lying on the positive side of a surface element (the side on the positive side of the outer normal) exerts on the part lying on the negative side. Stress is a tensor quantity. A normal stress is perpendicular to the surface while shear stress is parallel to the surface.
Turbulence	Turbulent flow is characterized by that the inertia stresses dominate over the viscous stresses, leading to small-scale chaotic behavior in the fluid motion.
Viscoelasticity	Time dependence of the response to stress and strain. Stress relaxation, creep and hysteresis are viscoelastic features.
Viscosity	The property of resisting deformation in a fluid. Viscosity relates the magnitude of fluid shear stresses to the fluid strain rate.
Zero-stress state	The tissue configuration when neither external nor internal forces are present. For tubular organs, the zero-stress state is assessed by making a radial cut in a tissue ring so that it springs open into a sector.

External forces from the environment of the gastrointestinal tract must be distinguished from the forces it generates itself. External forces that are applied to a gastrointestinal segment, both those from the outside and those from the lumen make it deform while, at the same time, it resists those forces. It has been a common practice to use compliance (and slightly more complex distensibility measures) to describe both the deformation and the resistance to deformation. Nevertheless, careful definition of these parameters can be difficult for the gastrointestinal tract since no single parameter can describe the complex mechanical behavior of the system. It is important to understand the concepts of stress and strain and the meaning of the constitutive equation to arrive at useful approximations. Fig. (**1**) illustrates the basic geometry of a cylindrical segment of the gastrointestinal tract. The three principal directions, circumferential (θ), longitudinal (z), and radial (r) are illustrated. The pressure caused by a bolus or a distending bag induces a normal stress that will stretch the tube in circumferential directions and likely also cause longitudinal extension and radial contraction, resulting in that the wall becomes thinner. If the pressure is generated by a moving bolus, longitudinal forces will also occur, resulting in mucosal shear stress. Normal stresses and shear stresses with their corresponding strains will be dealt with below.

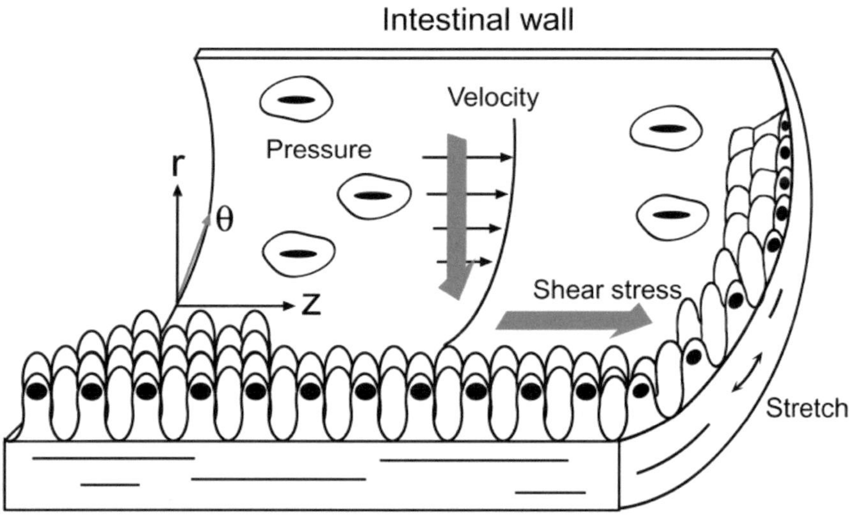

Figure 1: A schematic drawing of the intestinal wall. The circumferential, longitudinal, and radial directions are symbolized by θ, z, and r. The distension pressure induces normal stress that will stretch the tube in the circumferential direction and cause radial compression (a thinner wall). Longitudinal extension may occur. In addition a moving bolus will cause mucosal shear stresses (Modified from [16]).

2.3.2. Stress

The word "stress" has many meanings. Here we will consider only mechanical stress.

Consider a large and a small specimen. The small specimen can only sustain a small force whereas the large specimen can sustain a larger force. Hence, the force relative to the size is important. Stress is force per unit cross-sectional area ($\sigma = \frac{F}{A}$) with Pa or Nm^{-2} units (the SI unit for force is the Newton, the force required to give a mass of one kilogram an acceleration of 1 m s^{-2}). Force can be applied perpendicular to the surface, representing bolus pressure (normal stress) exerted on the wall, or parallel to the surface, representing force exerted by the fluid flow (shear stress) on the wall. Normal stresses may be either tensile or compressive. Forces can be applied in any direction and can induce stresses and strains in any direction. The state of stress at any given point in the body is described by a stress tensor consisting of three normal stresses and six shear stresses. This book does not intend to make use of tensor analysis but it is important to keep in mind the concept. This book primarily deals with derivation of equations for simple geometric structures based on equilibrium equations. One of the simplest equations to be used is La Place's law. The reader is referred to Fung for further reading on tensors [7, 24].

2.3.2.1. Stresses in Membranes and Shells

The law of Laplace has often been used in cardiovascular and gastrointestinal physiology because of its simplicity to explain why rupture occurs when segments of viscera are excessively distended. An important implication is that wall stress relates to pressure and to the wall thickness-to-radius ratio. Quantitative statements about such descriptive wall properties as distensibility, tone and the threshold for a mechanoreceptor response make no sense without consideration of the wall thickness-to-radius ratio (see later).

It is important to recognize the assumptions Laplace's law is based on. It was developed originally to describe the mechanical features of a homogeneous material with a simple geometry, *i.e.* the relationship between pressure, the curvature of a liquid surface, and surface tension. It was probably never meant to be used in physiology but nevertheless it receives attention from many investigators in gastrointestinal physiology. Two assumptions apply in respect to the law of Laplace for any tubular organ: the segment must geometrically be a circular cylinder with a uniform thickness in the entire circumference, and static equilibrium of forces is required. These conditions are virtually never met in physiology.

It is debatable whether the gastrointestinal tract can be regarded as thick-walled or thin-walled. This is of importance since one cannot assume stress to be uniform through the wall thickness in thick-walled cylinders. The limit is often considered to be at a wall thickness-to-radius ratio of 10% (hence, there is less than a 5% difference in the stress distribution from the inner to outer wall surface). The heart, arteries and arterioles have wall thickness-to-radius ratios of 0.25, 0.20 and 1.0. Consequently they must be modeled as thick-walled shells. The corresponding value for veins is 0.03. Hence, veins can be regarded as being thin-walled. Nevertheless, thin-walled stress theory has often been employed for other parts of the cardiovascular system, and justified by the assumption that the average stress is a reasonable approximation.

For the gastrointestinal tract, very few data has been published on the wall thickness-to-radius ratio. The esophagus is collapsed and buckles at the inner surface, hence, it has especially at low pressures a very high wall thickness-to-radius ratio (Fig. **2**). The small intestine, except the ileum, must likely be considered thick-walled. It is reasonable to consider the large intestine to be a thin-walled organ.

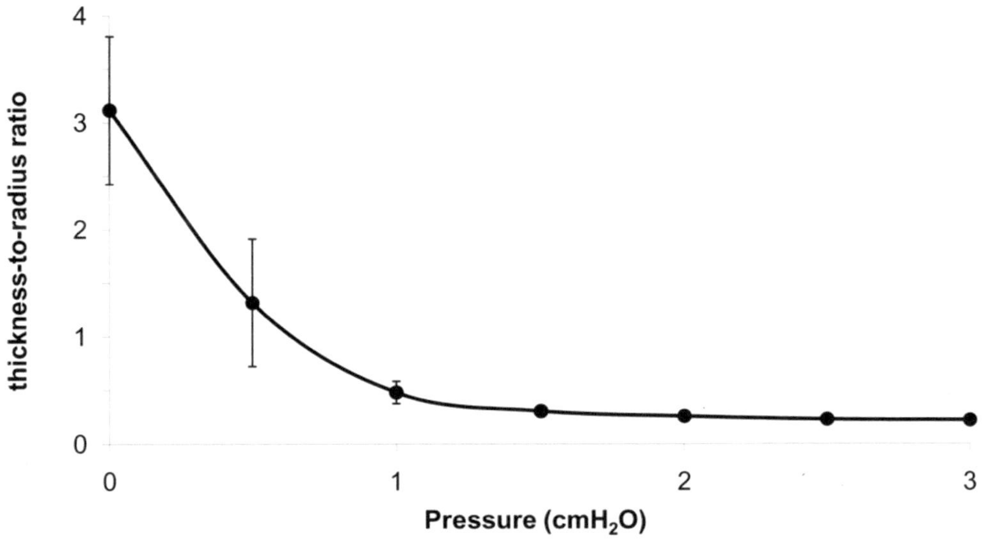

Figure 2: Data on the wall thickness-to-radius ratio for rat esophagus as function of pressure (courtesy of Professor Zhao).

2.3.2.2. Stresses in Thin-Walled Tubular Organs

First assume that the gastrointestinal tract is a thin-walled cylindrical pressure tube and that the weight of the gastrointestinal segment and contents inside can be neglected. In a cylindrical tube, we consider circumferential, longitudinal and radial components of stress in the respective directions. These are the normal components of stress in the cylinder wall (Fig. **3a**). Also additional shear components exit. We shall consider the circumferential stress, also named the hoop stress, and the longitudinal stress, also named the axial stress.

The major tensile stress induced by distension is in the circumferential direction in tubular organs. The equilibrium condition during luminal pressure loading requires the force in the circumferential direction in the wall to be balanced by the force contributed by the inflation pressure in the lumen. With cylindrical geometry, the average circumferential wall stress is

$$\tau_\theta = \frac{pr_i}{h} \tag{2.1}$$

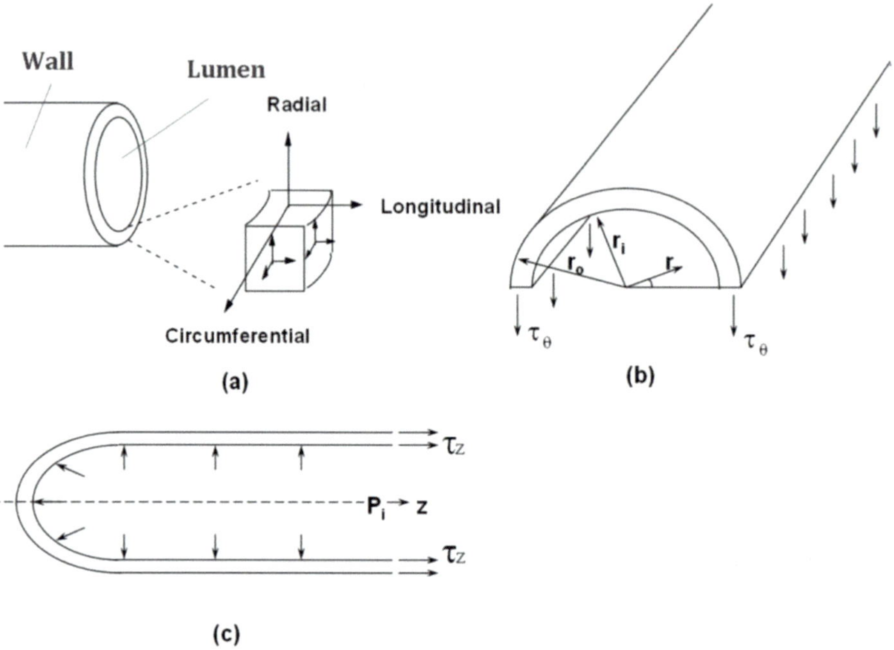

Figure 3: A pressurized cylindrical tube. **(a)** An infinitesimal element of the cylindrical tube showing the circumferential, longitudinal and radial directions. **(b)** A free-body diagram of half of the tube cut parallel to the central axis. **(c)** A free-body diagram of a tube cut perpendicular to the central axis (Modified from [17]).

where p, r_i, and h are the transmural pressure, internal radius, and wall thickness, respectively. This equation is commonly known as Laplace's law and it can be derived from consideration of equilibrium in the following way.

Consider a cylindrical intestine subjected to an internal pressure p_i, as shown in Fig. (**3a-c**). The luminal pressure induces wall stress. The external pressure is considered zero (but in reality it is not which may induce errors as pointed out by Brasseur and coworkers [25]). At equilibrium, the force in the circumferential direction in the wall $2\tau_\theta(r_o - r_i)L$, is balanced by the force in the lumen contributed by the pressure $2Lr_ip_i$ (Fig. **3b**). Hence, under equilibrium conditions $2\tau_\theta(r_o - r_i)L = 2Lr_ip_i$ and the equilibrium in the circumferential direction is expressed as

$$\tau_\theta = \frac{pr_i}{r_o - r_i} \tag{2.2}$$

where τ_θ is circumferential stress, r_i is internal radius and r_o is outer radius. Because $r_o - r_i = h$ = wall thickness, then Eq. 2.2 is simplified to Eq. 2.1. Note that the stress in Eq. 2.1 is averaged over the wall thickness and does not represent any stress distribution across the wall thickness. Furthermore, the Laplace stress may either refer to the wall thickness in the undeformed state (h_0) (called the *engineering stress*) or to the deformed state thickness *(true stress)*. For conical geometry as may occur in the stomach, the *circumferential stress* is given by Nash as [26]

$$\tau_\theta = \frac{pr_i}{h\cos\alpha} \tag{2.3}$$

where α represent the angle between the center line axis and wall of the cone. When α is small, Eq. 2.3 reduces to Eq. 2.1. When the deformation is expressed as a Green strain (large deformation theory (Lagrangian description, see later)), the stress must be expressed as a commensurate measure and in that case as a Kirchhoff stress

$$S_\theta = \frac{\Pr_i}{h\,\lambda_\theta^2} \tag{2.4}$$

where λ is the circumferential stretch ratio (circumferential length when the segment is pressurized divided by the circumferential length when unloaded). The Kirchhoff stress is useful in bi-axial strain energy functions with uniform $S_{\theta\theta}$ *and* S_{zz} (see later).

2.3.2.3. Stress in Thick-Walled Tubular Organs

If the organ is thick-walled, the stresses should not be averaged over the thickness. According to the solution by Lamé under the hypotheses of linearized theory for elasticity, the circumferential distribution of stress across the circular cylinder can be computed as

$$\sigma_\theta = \frac{r_o^2 r_i^2 (p_o - p_i)}{r^2 (r_o^2 - r_i^2)} + \frac{p_i r_i^2 - p_0 r_o^2}{r_o^2 - r_i^2} \tag{2.5a}$$

where r_0 and r_i are outer and inner radii, whereas r is the radial location of a point in the wall. p_0 and p_i are the outside and inside pressures. Consider an example of a segment with outer and inner radii of 7 and 5 mm and with a pressure in the lumen and an outer pressure of 0 kPa. Then the circumferential stress can be computed as function of the radius in the wall as shown in Fig. (**4**) for three pressure levels. It is clearly seen in the figure that the stress is highest at the inner surface and drops throughout the wall. The radial stress distribution can be computed in a similar fashion. The following equation is for the radial stress:

$$\sigma_r = \frac{r_o^2 r_i^2 (p_o - p_i)}{r^2 (r_o^2 - r_i^2)} + \frac{p_i r_i^2 - p_0 r_o^2}{r_o^2 - r_i^2} \tag{2.5b}$$

The thick-walled approach is best if one wants to determine the stress in the vicinity of the mechanoreceptors in the gastrointestinal wall. This accounts especially for the thick-walled esophagus. However, at least two important considerations must be made. First, a physiological mechanism exists to reduce the gradient in stress through the wall. Residual stress and strain (prestress) exist in the gastrointestinal tract. This can easily be demonstrated by a gastrointestinal segment opening into a sector when cut radially. If a cylinder is not prestressed, then it will bear the highest tensile stress at the inner edge (as shown in Fig. (**4**)) which will further increase during loading since the radius-wall thickness ratio increases. However, residual strain in biological tissues serves under homeostatic conditions to reduce the stress gradient from the inner wall to the outer wall (Chapter 4). Hence, residual strain prevents mucosal damage in the gastrointestinal tract during large bolus transport. Second, the gastrointestinal tract is layered with different mechanical properties for each layer. This phenomenon makes mechanical studies much more complicated and speaks in favor of the use of layered models for analysis of gastrointestinal mechanical function [16, 17].

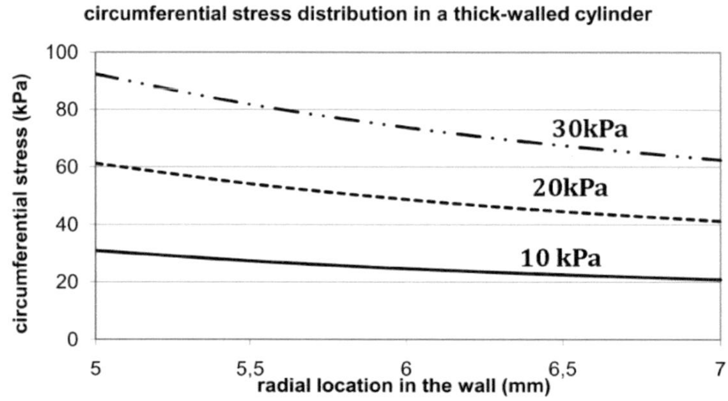

Figure 4: The distribution of circumferential stress computed according to thick-walled theory. In this example, the inner pressure is 10, 20 and 30 kPa and the inner and outer radii are 5 and 7 mm. The thick-walled approach considers the non-linear distribution in the wall and shows that the highest stress is found at the inner surface.

The wall longitudinal stress can be determined in a way similar to that for calculation of the circumferential stress, *i.e.* based on the equilibrium of forces in the longitudinal direction. The product of the cross-sectional area of the intestinal wall and the longitudinal stress is the force that balances the total longitudinal force acting on the intestine, as shown in Fig. (**3c**).

The longitudinal force in the wall $\tau_z\pi(r_o^2 - r_i^2)$ is balanced only by the pressure component $P_i\pi r_i^2$ since the external pressure is assumed to be zero. Thus, $\tau_z\pi(r_o^2 - r_i^2) = P_i\pi r_i^2$ and the longitudinal stress τ_z can be expressed as:

$$\tau_z = \frac{\mathrm{P}r_i^2}{r_o^2 - r_i^2} \qquad (2.6)$$

If the wall thickness-to-radius ratio is small, then $r_o = r_i = r$ and $r_o - r_i = h$, and the equation for longitudinal stress is simplified to

$$\tau_z = \frac{\mathrm{P}r_i}{2h} \qquad (2.7)$$

2.3.2.4. Stress (Tension) in a Membrane

Many readers will better know the following formulas as Laplace's law. The organ is considered to be very thin-walled and membrane theory must be considered rather than the abovementioned shell theory. Furthermore, tension is computed rather than stress. This approach is often used in physiological studies id the wall thickness is not measured or known.

Laplace's law originally refers to the relationship between the pressure difference, the curvature of the membrane surface, and the wall tension. If we consider a thin-walled membrane surface and make the assumption that the wall tension is constant everywhere, then the law of Laplace states

$$\mathrm{T} = \Delta\mathrm{P}\left(\frac{1}{r_1} + \frac{1}{r_2}\right)^{-1} \qquad (2.8)$$

where ΔP is the transmural pressure difference, r_1 and r_2 are the principal radii of the surface curvature, and T is the total tension per unit length of the mid-surface of the membrane. ΔP is equal to the pressure inside the membrane with the assumption that the external pressure is zero. In the case of cylindrical geometry, the equation reduces to T = ΔP r since one of the radii tends to infinity. For spherical geometry to T = $\Delta P \frac{r}{2}$ since the two radii in that case are equal. Laplace's law is often used for distension studies in tubular organs if the wall thickness is unknown. Other equations have to be considered if the luminal cross-sectional area is not circular but elliptical.

Eq. 2.8 is valid for membranes so thin that bending rigidity can be neglected. In addition, several underlying assumptions exist such as that the analysis requires a static equilibrium of forces and, consequently, zero inertial forces. Also as pointed out by Brasseur, the outside pressure cannot be considered to be zero [25]. The circumferential tension is the product of the wall thickness and the average circumferential stress (Eq. 2.1). Tension is also named the membrane stress resultant.

Stress in membranes is further dealt with later in this chapter.

2.3.2.5. Spheroidal Organs

The free-body diagram for the spheroidal geometry is shown in Fig. (**5**). In a similar way as for the longitudinal direction of a pressurized tube, the force in the wall of a thin-walled sphere $\tau_z\pi(r_o^2 - r_i^2)$ is balanced only by the pressure component $P_i\pi r_i^2$. With the abovementioned assumptions, Eq. 2.7 also applies to the thin-walled pressurized spherical shell.

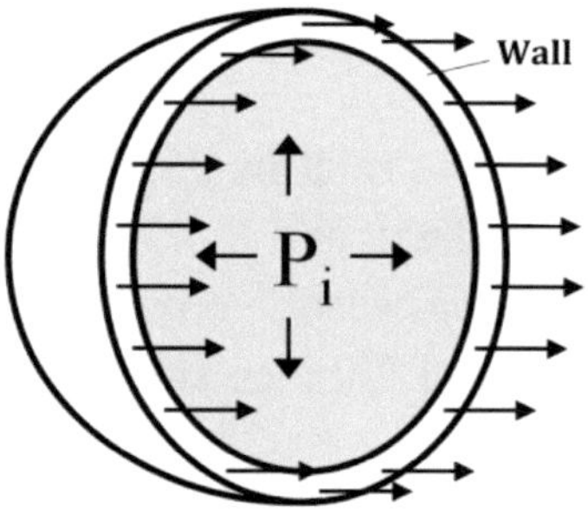

Figure 5: A free-body diagram of the pressurized spherical shell.

2.3.2.6. Determination of the Circumferential and Longitudinal Components of Membrane Tension during Bag Distension

Bag distension (by some called balloon distension) is a commonly used technique in visceral organs. Research studies often take advantage of this technique in the study of organ physiology. For example, investigators often use bag distension in the investigation of the force-deformation relationship and the activity of those neural sensory receptors that respond to mechanical stimulation. Bag distension is also used for diagnostic and therapeutic purposes. Examples include the diagnosis of non-cardiac chest pain, the ablation of plaques in coronary atherosclerosis, the compression of bleeding esophageal varices in liver disease, and dilatation of the lower esophageal sphincter in achalasia.

In a biomechanical analysis, it is important to know the force-deformation (stress-strain) relationship of the tissue. If the wall thickness is measurable and the intestine remains in cylindrical shape, then the average stress in the tissue can be determined according to Laplace's law as outlined above. However, the thickness is often not measurable and the shape of the bag-distended intestine is not exactly a cylinder. Then the force exerted on the tissue is expressed in terms of tension, and Laplace's law must be improved to remove the cylindrical shape restriction.

The theory outlined below can be used in any hollow visceral organ *in vitro* or *in vivo* as long as the geometric data and the bag pressure can be measured. The framework is developed for determination of the circumferential and longitudinal components of tension during bag distension. The basic message is that when we know the shape of the intestine, we can compute the circumferential and longitudinal components of tension. Bending forces and moments are neglected. It is assumed that the bag and intestine form a tube of revolution, that the structure and deformation are axisymmetric, that the zero-stress state of the bag has a diameter larger than that of the distended intestine and that its length is sufficiently longer than the intestinal segment in contact with the bag. The intestine resists the pressure imposed by the distending bag. We assume also that the friction (shear stress) between the bag and the intestine is negligible which probably requires lubrication of the bag surface. At places where the bag is in contact with the intestine during distension, we treat the tissue and bag together as a membranous structure. Coordinates are used as shown in Fig. (**6**), with z as the longitudinal axis, r as radial axis, θ the polar angle, and ϕ as the latitudinal angle. θ and ϕ form a set of curvilinear orthogonal coordinates. Membrane stress resultants are N_θ, N_ϕ, the circumferential and longitudinal membrane stresses, respectively. Definitions of these coordinates and stress resultants are given in the legend to Fig. (**6**) For an oversized bag we can assume that $N_\theta = N_\phi = 0$ for the bag.

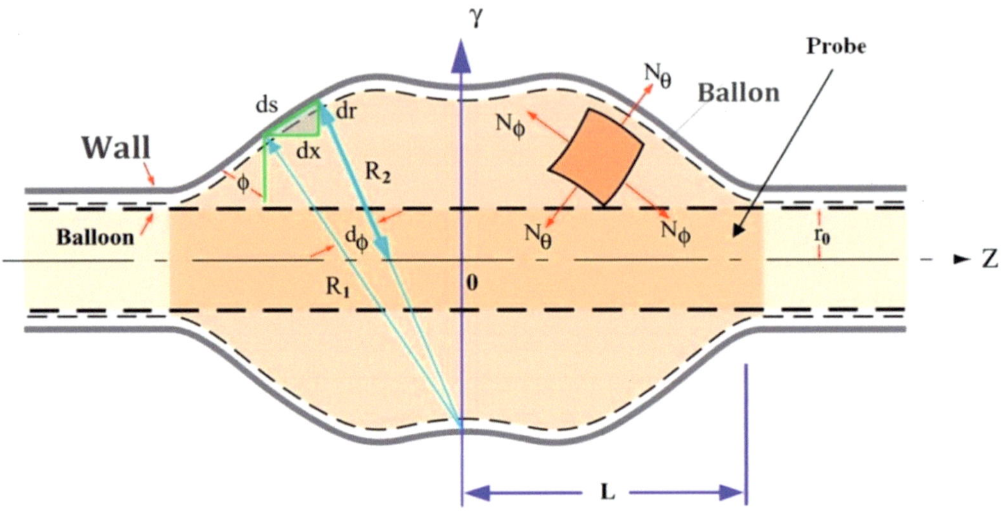

Figure 6: Geometry of the bag (balloon)-distended gastrointestinal segment. Two systems of coordinates are convenient: (1) the 3-dimensional cylindrical polar coordinates (r, θ, z). (2) the two-dimensional latitude-longitude coordinates (ϕ, θ) on the surface of the intestine. The latitudinal angle ϕ is defined as the angle between the normal vector to the surface of the intestine and the axis of symmetry z. The longitudinal angle θ is the angle of rotation of the meridional cross-section about the z axis. A normal vector exists at any point P on the surface with coordinate ϕ and θ. At a point near P, with coordinates (ϕ+dϕ and θ) another normal vector exists. These normal vectors will intersect at a distance r_1 from the surface. This r_1 is *a principal radius of curvature of the surface* in the longitudinal cross-section. On the other hand, the normals at (ϕ, θ) and (ϕ+dθ and θ) will intersect at a distance r_2 from the surface. r_2 is also a principal radius of curvature of the surface. The radius of curvature of the curve of intersection of any other normal plane at P lies between r_1 and r_2. Hence, the curvature of the intestinal surface is defined by r_1 and r_2.
The stresses of interest in an axi-symmetric tube subjected to axi-symmetric load are those lying in the wall, acting on normal cross-sections of the wall. A rectangular element with sides dϕ and dθ is shown. The stresses $\sigma_{\phi\phi}$ and $\sigma_{\theta\theta}$ can be much larger than the pressure in the bag, p. When the shear stress between the bag and intestine is ignored, and the bending stresses are ignored because the intestinal wall thickness is small compared with the radii of curvature, then $\sigma_{\phi\phi}$ and $\sigma_{\theta\theta}$ are uniformly distributed throughout the intestinal wall. Multiplying the uniform stresses $\sigma_{\phi\phi}$ and $\sigma_{\theta\theta}$ by the wall thickness, h, we obtain $N_\phi = \sigma_{\phi\phi}$ h and $N_\phi = \sigma_{\theta\theta}$ h which are called *membrane tensions* in cross-sections whose normal vectors lie in the direction of ϕ and θ axes, respectively. The units of N_ϕ, N_ϕ are force per unit length, N/m, like those of surface tension, while the stresses have units N/m^2. N_ϕ, N_ϕ are by some called *stress resultants* or *membrane stress resultants* to recognize the fact that they are the integrals of stresses throughout the thickness of the membrane wall (Modified from [17] and MCB 2004).

The boundary condition for stress in the intestine is $N_\theta = 0 = N_\phi$ when $z \rightarrow \infty$. The shear $N_{\theta\phi}$ is zero for axisymmetric deformation. The radius of curvature of the longitudinal section is r_1. The radius of curvature of the intestinal surface in a normal section orthogonal to the longitudinal direction is r_2. Fig. (**6**) shows the following geometric relationships:

$$r = r_2 \sin \phi,\ ds = r_1\, d\phi \tag{2.9}$$

$$dz = r_1 \sin \phi\, d\phi,\ dr = r_1 \cos \phi\, d\phi \tag{2.10}$$

The equations of equilibrium are

$$\frac{N_\varphi}{r_1} + \frac{N_\theta}{r_2} = p\ , \tag{2.11}$$

$$\frac{d}{d\phi}(r\,N_\phi) - r_1\, N_\theta \cos\phi = 0 \tag{2.12}$$

where p is the pressure in the bag.

Solving Eq. 2.11 for N_θ and substituting the result into Eq. 2.12 and reducing, we obtain

$$\frac{d}{d\phi}(rN_\phi) + r_2 \cos\phi N_\phi - pr_1 r_2 \cos\phi = 0 \tag{2.13}$$

On multiplying by sin ϕ and using Eq. 2.9, we obtain

$$\frac{d}{d\varphi}(r_2 N_\varphi \sin^2\varphi) = pr_1 r_2 \cos\varphi \sin\varphi \tag{2.14}$$

Hence,

$$N_\varphi = \frac{1}{r_2 \sin^2\varphi} \int pr_1 r_2 \cos\varphi\ \sin\varphi\ d\varphi \tag{2.15}$$

Using the geometric relationships in Eqs. 2.9 and 2.10, we obtain

$$N_\varphi = \frac{1}{r \sin\varphi} \int_{r_o}^{r} pr\,dr = \frac{p(r^2 - r_o^2)}{2r\sin\varphi} \tag{2.16}$$

where r_o is an integration constant. Since N_ϕ tends to zero when $z \to \infty$, we see that r_o is the radius of intestine sufficiently far away from the bag. An alternative expression for N_ϕ as a function of z is:

$$N_\varphi = \frac{1}{r \sin\varphi}\left[p\int_0^z r_2 \cos\varphi \; dz + C \right] \tag{2.17}$$

where C is an integration constant.

If at a large distance $z = L_o$, $r = r_{Lo}$, $\phi=\pi/2$, $N_\phi = N_\phi^{(\infty)}$, total longitudinal force = 2 $\pi\, r_\infty\, N_\phi^{(\infty)} = T$, then

$$T = 2\pi\left[p\int_0^{L_o} r_2 \cos\varphi \, dz + C \right] \tag{2.18}$$

Of special interest is the case in which T = 0, *i.e.* where the longitudinal tension in the intact intestine is zero. Then

$$C = -p\int_0^{L_o} r_2 \cos\varphi \, dz \tag{2.19}$$

With this C, we can then compute the value of $N_\phi^{(0)}$. This gives the longitudinal tensile stress resultant N_ϕ at the centre section $z = 0$

Using Eq. 2.16 or Eq. 2.17 in Eq. 2.11, we have

$$\mathrm{N}_\theta = r_2\left(p - \frac{N_\varphi}{r_1}\right) \tag{2.20}$$

Combining with Eqs. 2.16 or 2.17 we obtain

$$N_\theta = r_2 \,\mathrm{p}\left(1 - \frac{r^2 - r_o^2}{2 r r_1 \sin\varphi}\right) \tag{2.21}$$

Hence, if the radii of curvature r_1, r_2 are measured from a photograph of the intestinal profile, then the membrane stress resultants N_θ, N_ϕ can be computed everywhere in the part of the intestine that is in contact with the bag.

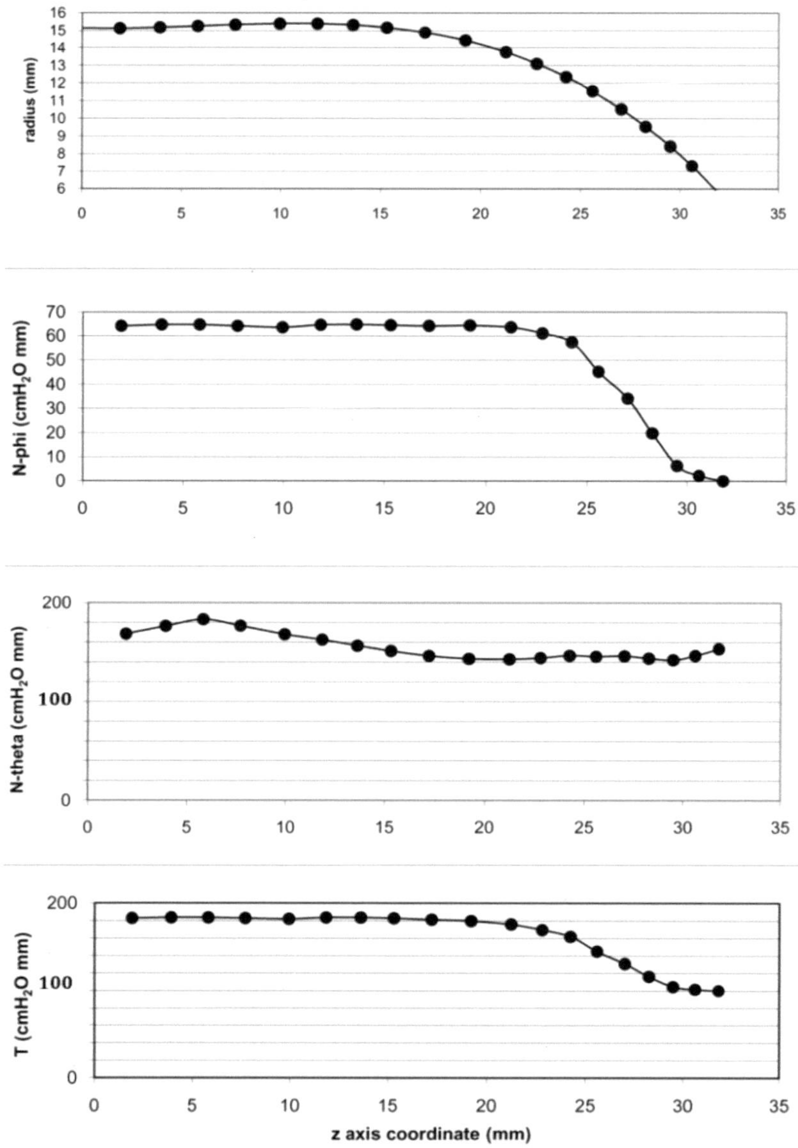

Figure 7: Representation of radii, N_ϕ, N_θ and T_L obtained at pressure levels up to 12 cmH_2O as function of z for a pig experiments. N_ϕ and T_L are seen to resemble the shape of the radii, whereas N_θ has a local maximum 20-30% away from the middle of the bag (Modified from [17] and MCB 2004).

Fig. (**7**) shows the radius, N_ϕ, N_θ and T_L obtained by this method from the intestine in 40-kg pigs at a bag pressure of 12 cm H_2O as function of z (the tension T_L was computed according to Laplace's law, $T_L = p\ r$ for comparison with N_θ). From the figure it appears that N_ϕ increases with the pressure, is highest at the mid-bag location, and decreases towards the end of the bag. N_θ also increases with the pressure applied and is, in general, 2-3 times higher than N_ϕ. At the highest pressure applied, the maximum N_θ is located approximately 25% away from the middle of the bag.

T_L exceeds N_θ from 0% to about 70% away from the middle of the bag. Only at the location of maximal N_θ are N_θ and T_L similar. At about 80% away from the middle of the bag, N_θ becomes higher than T_L. The longitudinal tension (N_ϕ) and T_L behave much as expected, with maximum values at the middle of the bag. However, N_θ has its maximum approximately 25% away from the middle of the bag. The reason for this conformation of the intestine during distension lacks an explanation but energy considerations may be important. The analysis indicates that tension computed directly from Laplace's law does not provide very accurate measures of circumferential tension.

The theory presented can be applied to the organ that is situated *in vivo* as long as the shape and the pressure can be obtained. The technique of bag distension with pressure-volume measurement cannot provide such data. However, there are several other ways to obtain the data *in vivo*. Impedance planimetry can provide measures of the bag cross-sectional area at various locations on the z-axis (in recent years named the functional luminal imaging probe (FLIP) technology) and, assuming circularity, the internal radii can be computed. X-ray is another way to provide the geometric data. Furthermore, B-mode ultrasound or 3D-ultrasound, multi-slice CT-scanning and MR scanning can all provide a three-dimensional profile of the distended area. Another advantage with these techniques is that the wall thickness can be measured. Hence, the stress rather than the tension can be computed in the two directions. For the ultimate *in vivo* application, such aspects as the determination of the transmural pressure difference (solutions are presented in Gregersen and Kassab 1996 [17]), the resolution and sensitivity of the method used, tethering between organs, and similar considerations all need to be evaluated and errors need to be estimated.

The strain analysis can be implemented in a similar fashion as the stress analysis. Assuming that the constitutive equation for the intestine is similar to that of other soft tissues, then the full non-linear constitutive equation can be derived.

It is of considerable interest to obtain the three-dimensional (3-D) geometry of visceral organs. Fourier series analysis has been developed to describe the surfaces of the stomach and rectum and to transform the geometry from a 3-D

Cartesian coordinate to a 2-D local tangent plane coordinate system [18, 21]. The geometric data can then be used to compute the tension and stress using Laplace's equation under conditions for a thin-walled structure. A geometric reconstruction of the human stomach from 3D ultrasonography is shown in Fig. (**8**).

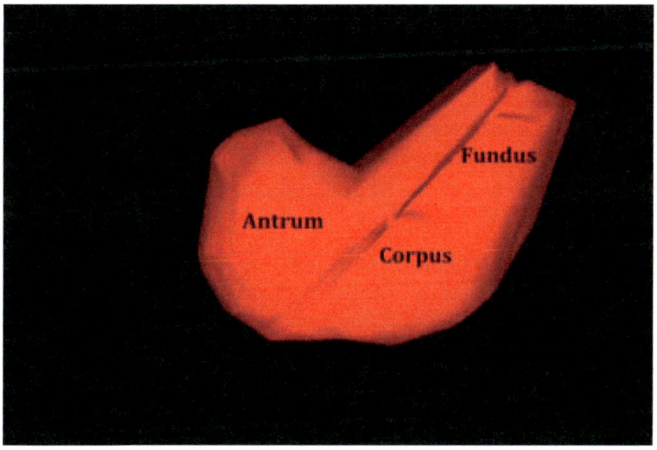

Figure 8: Geometric reconstruction of the human stomach based on 3D ultrasound data. [The figure is kindly provided by Dr. Odd Helge Gilja, Bergen, Norway].

2.3.3. Strain and Strain Rate

"Deformation" is a term referring to a change in the shape of a continuum between an initial undeformed configuration and a subsequent deformed configuration. Deformation can occur in many ways. Examples are stretch of a strip of tissue when we pull it, and distension of a tubular organ when we pressurize the lumen. The strain measures are useful for description of such deformations quantitatively. Force can be applied in any direction and may induce strains in any direction. The strain may be perpendicular to the surface which is called normal strain, or it may be parallel to the surface also called shear strain. The latter is for example the strain exerted on the wall of a viscus by the flow of fluid. The state of strain at any given point in the body is described by a strain tensor consisting of three normal strains and six shear strains (as shown in Fig. (**2**) for stress). Three of the shear strains are independent. Strain rate is a change in strain as function of time, in other words the derivative of the strain-time curve.

2.3.3.1. Strain Measures

For a continuum being deformed, strains can be defined in relation to the deformation gradient in several ways. First, consider a strip of tissue of initial length L_0 (Fig. **9**).

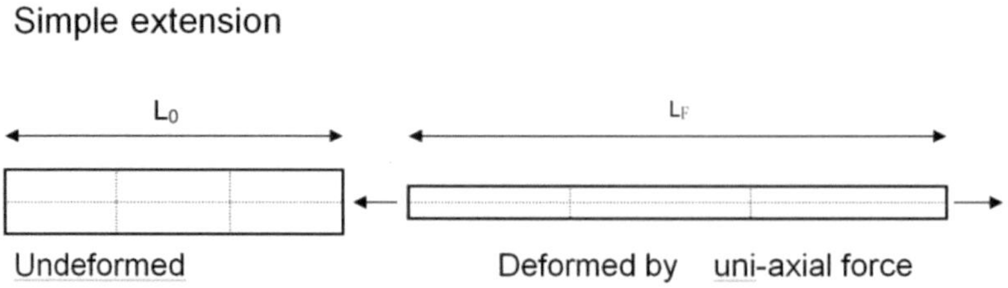

Figure 9: Extension of a strip (bar) with un-deformed length (L_0) at resting state and deformed length L caused by a uni-axial force. The force induces a tensile (positive) strain. A compressive (negative) strain is induced by a force in the opposite direction.

Stretching it to length L, the length change can be described by dimensionless ratios such as

$$\text{Stretch ratio } \lambda = \frac{L}{L_0} \tag{2.22}$$

$$\text{Cauchy strain } \in = \frac{L - L_0}{L_0} \tag{2.23}$$

$$\text{Green's strain E} = \frac{L^2 - L_0^2}{2L_0^2} \tag{2.24}$$

Hence, strains can be defined in different ways in relation to the deformation gradient for a continuum subjected to finite deformation. Selection of the proper strain measure is dictated primarily by the stress-strain relationship. The strains can be computed for all surfaces or interfaces between layers where the needed geometric data can be obtained. These measures are all dimensionless which is advantageous since the absolute length and any system of units are eliminated from consideration. This makes comparison easy between specimens of various sizes. In Eqs. 2.22-2.24, the strain measures are expressed as fractions of the initial length. Such strains are called Lagrangian strains. However, strains can also be expressed as fraction of the final length; in this case they are called Eulerian strains. Both Lagrangian and Eulerian strains measures are useful. In very small (infinitesimal) elongations, the strain measures are equal. However, in large (finite) elongations, they are different which easily can be demonstrated. The Cauchy strain is useful in the linearized elasticity theory, which is valid when $\in$ is infinitesimal. Hence, it is often called the "engineering strain" or "infinitesimal strain". Strain defined by Green is more conveniently related to stress for finite deformations. The strain measures can be transformed into another as shown below:

$$\in = \lambda - 1 \text{ and } E = \frac{(\in + 1)^2 - 1}{2} \qquad (2.25)$$

At this point, we may learn more about deformation from the experimental stretch of a strip of tissue. Because of the incompressible nature of tissue, stretching the strip causes radial narrowing which also is called lateral contraction. Thus, deformation in one direction causes deformation in other directions. In a body under tensile or compressive forces the ratio of lateral strain to longitudinal strain is called Poisson's ratio. Poisson's ratio is often regarded as 0.5 for biological materials since they are regarded as incompressible in the physiological range.

In some cases one strain measure may have advantages over others. As stated previously, Green strain and Kirchhoff stress are commensurate measures useful in strain energy functions. However, the stretch ratio is convenient when the tissue can be considered incompressible. The product of the stretch ratios in the three principal directions equals 1 if the tissue is incompressible. Hence, if two stretch ratios are known, it is possible to compute the last stretch ratio. For example, if the wall cross-sectional area is known, it is possible to compute the axial extension during mechanical loading, and if all three principal stretch ratios are known, the compressibility assumption can be tested. The proof is quite simple for this relation. A rectangular tissue block of tissue will have length L, width W, and height H and use the subscript 0 for the undeformed state. For the undeformed state the volume $V_0 = L_0\ W_0\ H_0$ and for the deformed state V = L W H. For incompressible tissue $V = V_0$. Therefore, $L_0\ W_0\ H_0$ = L W H or

$$\frac{L\,W\,H}{L_0\,W_0\,H_0} = 1 \text{ or } \lambda_L\lambda_W\lambda_H = 1 \qquad (2.26)$$

Soft biological tissues are characterized by that they, with a very low degree of compressibility, can undergo large deformations. Thus, biological tissues resist changes in volume much more than they resist changes in shape. Soft tissues can be considered incompressible for most practical applications within the physiological range. This has indeed been shown for arterial tissue but it remains an assumption in tissues from the gastrointestinal wall.

In this book, the focus is primarily on deformations caused by the application of luminal forces (pressure) in hollow organs like the intestines and esophagus. Bag distension is a controlled and physiological way of applying forces to the gastrointestinal tract wall. The rationale will be explained further in the chapters about smooth muscle function and residual strain.

As long as the geometric data can be obtained the strain measures can be used readily for investigating organs of complex configuration. For the gastrointestinal tract, we can for simplicity consider a tube of homogenous wall material that is straight circular and cylindrical. There will be circumferential, longitudinal and radial strain components as described above. These strains are the normal strain wall components. Distension by luminal pressure loading causes the circumferential length to increase (circumferential tensile strain), the wall thickness to decrease (radial compressive strain) and compression or elongation in the longitudinal direction (the material properties determines whether it is compressed or elongated). Contraction of the circumferential muscle layer will induce compressive (negative) circumferential wall strain and wall thickening.

An important issue in biomechanics is the determination of the initial length. Eqs. 2.22-2.24 clearly show that correct determination of the initial length is important for strain calculations. For several reasons it is a difficult task to determine the initial length. One reason is that suppression of smooth muscle activity can be difficult. Another reason is that strain likely vary throughout the intestinal wall. However, even more importantly, as outlined in later in this book, the zero-stress state can only be determined when the tissue is cut open, which obviously only is possible *in vitro*. When the strain is referred to the zero-stress state, the tissue is in tension when $\lambda > 1$. It is in compression when $\lambda < 1$. Tissue buckling occurs when $\lambda < 1$. Our assumption is that, for very soft tissucs in the neighborhood of a state of zero-stress or no-load, the critical buckling stress tends to zero. Esophagus, intestine and blood vessels probably belong to this category. Buckling is a global or macroscopic phenomenon. Hence the edge lengths E should be measured with a scale commensurate with the wall thickness of the tube, and not by fractal considerations.

Other methods are needed when the zero-stress state geometry cannot be obtained. Comparing strains and tension-strain relations for different segments or before and after interventions, r_0 may be evaluated at the same tension level in accordance with Laplace's law. In this way, a tension *versus* radius plot for each data set can be extrapolated to provide the lowest tension value. It is easy to determine r_0 graphically for the different specimens at this specific tension value. For ease of measurements, c and c_0, the corresponding circumferences, can replace r and r_0. Curve fitting is often needed. In that regard, numerous valid measurements points should be obtained as close to the unloaded state as possible. It should also be emphasized that the mid-wall radius should be determined for the determination of average stress-strain relations such as Cauchy strain and Cauchy stress using Laplace's law. Since such data may not be available from *in vivo* studies, we often see in many studies that the luminal radius is used.

Strain measures can be obtained in several ways. Let us first consider *In vitro* experiments. In this case strains are usually calculated from measurements of tissue strip length changes, from change in distance between surface or embedded tissue markers, or from the measurement of diameter changes in intact specimens. It is also often possible to determine the zero-stress state as the reference *in vitro*. For *in vivo* experiments bag distension techniques are often used with measurements of pressure, cross-sectional area or volume. When comparing experiments done *in vivo* with experiments done *in vitro*, it should be emphasized that the segments *in vitro* are often free to lengthen but *in vivo* they may be influenced by surrounding structures and even tethered to the surrounding structures. A good example of this is the observation that the esophagus *in vivo* is always exposed to a large longitudinal stress. It shortens up to 50% when removed from the body as observed in opossums and guinea pigs with a corresponding diameter increase. The large esophageal longitudinal strain and stress likely have physiological implications concerning bolus transport.

Twisting caused by torsional forces and bending may also be of importance in biomechanical studies of gastrointestinal function.

2.3.4. Constitutive Equations and Material Constants

Constitutive equations are used to describe material properties. In solid mechanics a constitutive equation relates stress and strain through a set of material constants. The *elastic modulus* is the proportionality constant between stress and strain. For a linear Hookean material this constant is called Young's modulus. For linear Hookean materials, the mechanical properties are elastic and the constitutive equation is simplified to Hooke's law. However, in soft biological tissues like the gastrointestinal tract, the strain is large (finite) and the stress-strain relation is non-linear. Gastrointestinal examples of large deformations and non-linear stress-strain relations are provided many places in this book. The non-linear mechanical behavior is often exponential, which reflects the mechanical properties of collagen and muscle. Nonlinear behavior facilitates stretch in the physiological pressure range and prevents overstretch and tissue damage at high stress levels. If the tissue is overstretched, then plastic deformation may occur. Plastic deformation is characterized by that the tissue can no longer return to its original state when unstressed. In tissues characterized by non-linear properties, it is necessary to compute an incremental elastic modulus or nonlinear constants. Biological tissues like the gastrointestinal wall possess complex three-dimensional structures that have different material properties in different directions. This important feature is called anisotropy and it implies that a large set of material constants have to be determined for complete description of the mechanical behavior.

Exponential or polynomial laws are often used to determine material constants. Stress-strain data are fitted using for example a least-square method with an exponential stress-strain relationship. A simple form can be expressed as

$$\sigma = \beta[\exp(\alpha\varepsilon) - 1] \tag{2.27}$$

With strain referenced to the zero-stress state, $\sigma = 0$ when $\varepsilon = 0$, as satisfied by Eq. 2.27. The values of α and β are usually determined by a least square fit for the circumferential and longitudinal directions. The tangent modulus, E, is defined as the slope of the stress-strain relationship and is a measure of tissue stiffness. It can be computed analytically from Eq. 2.27 as

$$E = \frac{d\sigma}{d\varepsilon} = \alpha[\sigma + \beta] \tag{2.28}$$

The tangent modulus is equivalent to Young's modulus in the linear stress-strain range. This equation was originally used in uni-axial strip experiments but it can be used independently for circumferential and longitudinal direction data obtained from distensions of gastrointestinal tract. It is however more correct to use a bi-axial approach which is given below.

Incremental elastic moduli can also be computed for nonlinear stress-strain relations. For comparison of these moduli, they must be measured at constant strains. Dobrin has provided cardiovascular examples of the error introduced in expressing such moduli as function of pressure and different length settings [27].

2.3.4.1. Biaxial Approach for the Analysis of Strain and Stress in the Gastrointestinal Wall

For quantifying wall stresses, both accurate measurement of the strain field to which the gastrointestinal tract is subjected and a reliable constitutive equation that relates those strains to stresses are necessary. Based on experience the gastrointestinal wall is exposed to finite deformation and can be assumed to be an incompressible, non-linearly elastic, orthotropic material. The use of a strain energy functions are convenient for which the strains are referenced to the zero-stress state. The strain energy function of the gastrointestinal wall represents stored energy per unit volume. One strain energy function in a two-dimensional analysis is expressed according to Fung as follows,

$$\rho_0 W = \frac{C}{2} e^Q \tag{2.29}$$

$$Q = a_1(E^2_{\theta\theta} - E^{*2}_{\theta\theta}) + a_2(E^2_{zz} - E^{*2}_{zz}) + 2a_4(E_{\theta\theta}\, E_{zz} - E^*_{\theta\theta}\, E^*_{zz})] \tag{2.30}$$

where P_0 is the material density (mass per unit volume), W is the strain energy per unit mass, P_0W is the strain energy per unit volume, and $E_{\theta\theta}$ and E_{ZZ} are the circumferential and longitudinal Green's strains. $E^*_{\theta\theta}$ and E^*_{ZZ} are reference strains measured at a physiological conditions, and C, a_1, a_2 and a_4 are material coefficients. If we assume that the wall material is homogeneous and pseudo elastic, *i.e.* the loading and unloading stress-strain curves are thought to represent properties of two materials with different elasticity, the strain energy function can be applied separately to the loading and unloading processes. The stress components can be expressed as

$$S_{ij} = \frac{\delta(\rho_0 W)}{\delta E_{ij}} \tag{2.31}$$

where S_{ij} and E_{ij} are components of Kirchhoff's stress and Green's strain. The homogeneity assumption can partly be tested in the case of esophagus by separating the layers of the esophagus and studying them independently. By combining Eqs. 2.29 and 2.31 and by neglecting any shear component, the stress-strain relations of a gastrointestinal segment can be obtained in both circumferential and longitudinal directions. The stress and strain components can be determined by experiment. The coefficients C, a_1, a_2 and a_4 of the strain energy function can be determined using non-linear curve-fitting methods.

The zero-stress state of the gastrointestinal segment at which the diameter and length are measured in the mechanical test, can be determined as described elsewhere in this book. The inner and outer wall circumferential lengths must be measured in the zero-stress state. The mid-wall circumferential length is calculated as

$$L_\theta = \frac{L_\theta^i + L_\theta^o}{2} \tag{2.32}$$

where L, L^i_θ and L^o_θ are the mid-, inner- and outer-wall circumferential lengths of the segment in the zero-stress state, respectively.

The mid-wall strain and average stress can be determined assuming that the material in the wall is homogenous and that the organ shape is cylindrical. The mid-wall circumferential strain can be computed from the measured outer diameters at varying pressure levels and from the zero-stress state mid-wall circumferential length. Assuming incompressible materials, the mid-wall circumferential length of the segment can be computed at a given inflation or deflation pressure when knowing the length and the outer diameter of the pressurized segment and the zero-stress state inner and outer wall circumference and longitudinal lengths. The mid-wall circumferential stretch ratio λ_θ can be computed at a given pressure as the ratio between the mid-wall circumferential length at a given pressurized state and the mid-wall circumferential length at the zero-stress state. In a similar way, the longitudinal stretch ratio λ_z can be computed at a given pressure as the ratio between the longitudinal length at a given pressure level and the longitudinal length in the zero-stress state. The circumferential and longitudinal Green strains ($E_{\theta\theta}$ and E_{zz}) and thc Kirchhoff stresses ($S_{\theta\theta}$ and S_{zz}) can be computed at a given pressure with the equations provided previously in this chapter.

The following stress-strain relations for the gastrointestinal segment in both the circumferential (θ) and longitudinal (z) directions can be obtained by substitution of Eq. 2.29 into Eq. 2.31,

$$S_{\theta\theta} = C(a_1E_{\theta\theta} + a_4E_{zz})e^Q \tag{2.33}$$

$$S_{zz} = C(a_2E_{zz} + a_4E_{\theta\theta})e^Q \tag{2.34}$$

The reference strains $E^*_{\theta\theta}$ and E^*_{zz} are selected at physiological pressures in the circumferential and longitudinal directions. The experimental data can be fitted using a Marquardt's non-linear least-squares algorithm. Furthermore, the C, a_1, a_2 and a_4 coefficients can be determined by minimizing the sum of the squares of the differences between experimental and theoretical data.

2.4. TIME-DEPENDENT (VISCOELASTIC) MECHANICAL PROPERTIES

Biological tissues exhibit both elastic solid and viscous fluid properties. Therefore, the stress depends not only on the applied strain but also on the rate of strain as in a viscous fluid. This means that the response is time-dependent, *i.e.* the stress-strain response does not occur instantly. After a sudden strain to a material and maintaining that strain constant, results in that the corresponding stresses induced in the wall decrease with time. This reflects a mechanical phenomenon called stress relaxation (Fig. **10**). Another phenomenon occurs when the material is suddenly stressed and the stress is maintained constant. In this case the material continues to deform. This phenomenon is called creep. A third phenomenon is when the material is subjected to a cyclic loading. In this case the stress-strain relationship in the unloading process is somewhat different from that in the loading process (Fig. **10**). This phenomenon is called hysteresis. Stress relaxation, creep and hysteresis are considered to be features of viscoelasticity.

The Maxwell model, the Voigt model and the Kelvin model (also called a standard linear solid) are three simple viscoelastic models often used. In these viscoelastic models linear springs (constant μ) are combined with dashpots with a coefficient of viscosity (η). The spring produces an instant deformation proportional to the load. In contrary the dashpot produces a velocity proportional to the load. The spring is described by the relationship $F = \mu u$, where F is a force acting on the spring and u is the extension of the spring. We have the relationship $F = \eta \dot{u}$ for the dashpot where $\dot{u}$ is the deflection velocity. The Maxwell body is the combination of a spring and dashpot in series. A spring and dashpot in parallel express the Voigt body and the Kelvin model has a dashpot in parallel with the Maxwell body. Creep functions and relaxation functions can be derived for these models on basis of the equations for the dashpot and spring. The creep behaviors for the three models are illustrated in Fig. (**11**). Though more complex viscoelastic functions exist, such models do not account for all history-dependent mechanical behavior as illustrated in section 2.5 about preconditioning and strain softening.

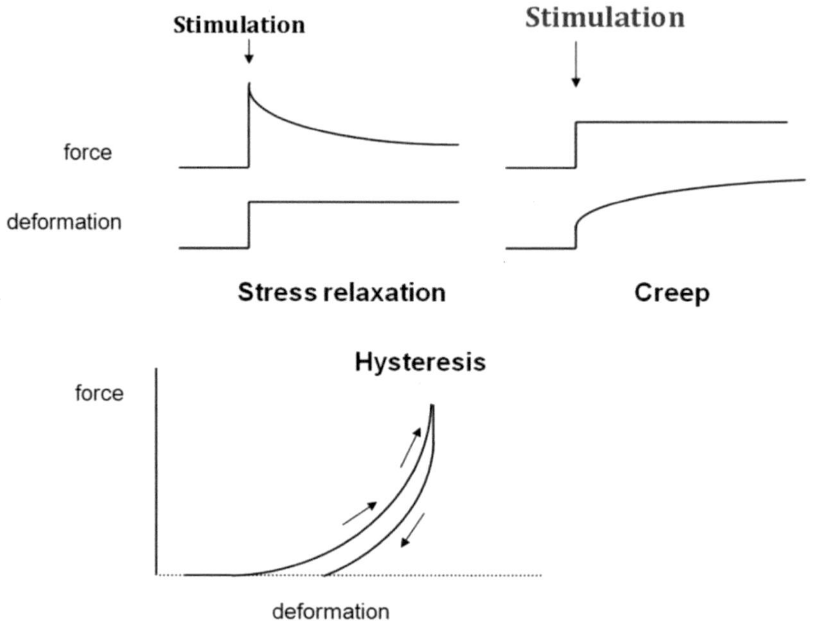

Figure 10: Illustration of stress relaxation, creep and hysteresis.

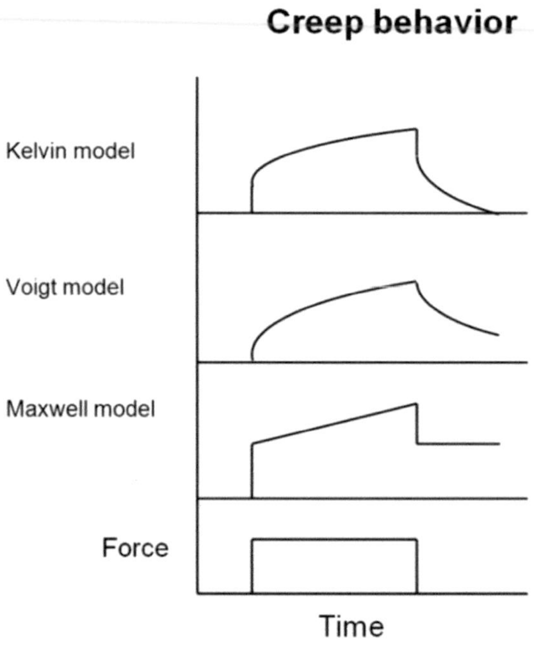

Figure 11: Illustration of the creep behavior in three viscoelastic models.

2.4.1. Modeling Creep Behavior using a Standard Linear Solid Model

Experimental creep data can be used to model the change as a function of time by fitting the observed data to the Kelvin model for a standard linear solid. Experimental data can be fitted to the exponential function

$$\theta(t) = \theta_0\left[1-\eta e^{-\lambda t}\right] \tag{2.35}$$

where

θ_o = asymptotic steady state value of the opening angle

λ = the creep rate (s^{-1})

t = time after the initial cut (s)

η = the creep fraction (non-dimensional)

This equation relates to the Kelvin body as follows. In the model, μ_1 and μ_2 are spring constants and η_1 is a coefficient of viscosity. If τ_ε = relaxation time for constant strain, τ_σ = relaxation time for constant stress and E_R = relaxed elastic modulus we can express

$$\tau_\varepsilon = \frac{\eta_1}{\mu_1},\ \tau_\sigma = \frac{\eta_1}{\mu_0}\left(1+\frac{\mu_0}{\mu_1}\right),\ E_R = \mu_0, \tag{2.36}$$

The equation describing this model can be obtained

$$C(t) = \frac{1}{E_R}\left[1-\left(1-\frac{\tau_\varepsilon}{\tau_\sigma}\right)e^{-\frac{t}{\tau_\sigma}}\right] \tag{2.37}$$

letting

$$\alpha = \frac{1}{E_R};\eta = 1-\frac{\tau_\varepsilon}{\tau_\sigma};\lambda = \frac{1}{\tau_\sigma} \tag{2.38}$$

The empirical constants η and λ can be used to plot predicted creep curves. The empirical constants α, η and λ can then be calculated.

2.5. PRECONDITIONING BEHAVIOR. STRAIN SOFTENING

In *in vitro* mechanical testing of living tissues, preconditioning is absolutely necessary for obtaining repeatable results. In preconditioning testing the specimen to be tested is mounted on the testing machine and loading and unloading processes are repeated until the stress-strain relationship becomes reproducible. The number of cycles required varies from one tissue to another with the method of preparation. Investigators in gastrointestinal studies often fail to pay attention to the importance of preconditioning, resulting in faulty results and erroneous conclusions. Fig. (**12**) shows an example of preconditioning behavior in the gastrointestinal tract. The repeatability and reproducibility of experiments made without preconditioning in studies both *in vitro* and *in vivo*: are not good. The rationale for preconditioning is that the tissues are disturbed during the tissue preparation by cutting, by changes in external stress and strain, temperature, blood flow, ischemia, hypoxia, chemical changes and contracture of muscle. Therefore the tissue needs to return to a stable condition by preconditioning. In most gastrointestinal tissues 3-10 cycles are needed before the tissue can be considered to be preconditioned. Conventional viscoelastic theory does not explain the adaptive changes that occur during preconditioning. A strain softening theory has been developed to explain it.

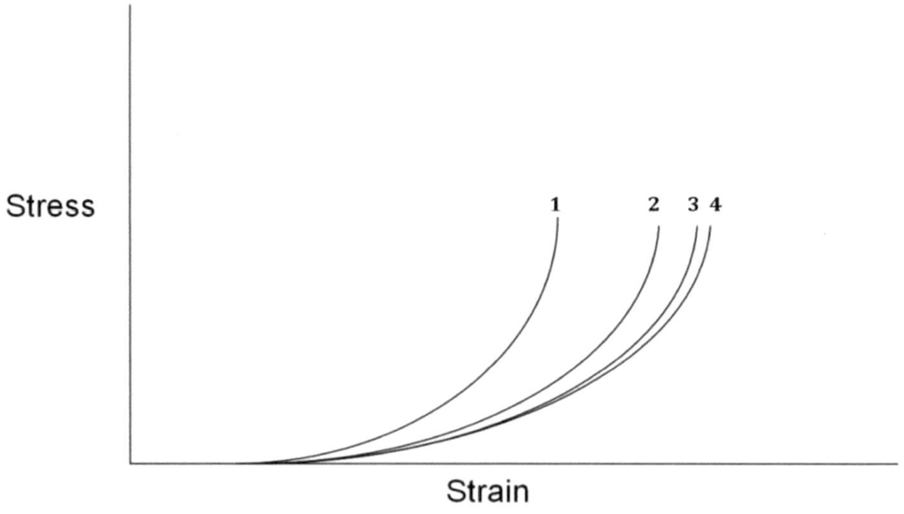

Figure 12: Demonstration of the preconditioning behavior. The stress-strain curve moves to the right until a stable condition is obtained. In the gastrointestinal tract it normally takes 3-4 loading cycles before the tissue is preconditioned.

Preconditioning is invariably associated with a loss of stiffness as the loading is repeated. The number of cycles depends on the tissue and the method of preparation. Preconditioning in soft tissues has conventionally been recognized as a viscoelastic property, in a similar way as creep and stress relaxation. However, certain rubber materials were found to exhibit different strain-history dependence. The stress-strain relation in rubber depends on the maximum previous load experienced. This property is now known as strain softening, or the Mullins effect. The fact that certain elastomers become permanently softened after the load reaches a new maximum for the first time has led to the suggestion, by Johnson and Beatty in 1993 [28], that strain softening may explain preconditioning behavior. Thus, some of the history dependence in soft tissues that has previously been attributed to viscoelasticity may actually be the result of strain softening. Emery and coworkers provided evidence in 1997 that the preconditioning behavior of the resting myocardium is due to strain softening and is relatively independent of the time-history of the load [29]. The passive properties of the tissue that depend on the time-history of load (viscoelastic effects) must be distinguished from those that depend on the maximum previous load (strain softening effects).

The preconditioning behavior (the changes that take place in preconditioning) of the jejunum is due largely to strain softening and is only weakly dependent on the time-history of loading. Gregersen and coworkers showed this in the isolated guinea-pig jejunum *in vitro* during cyclic inflation and deflation of a bag (approximately 10 inflation-deflation cycles) [30]. The strain softening effects in this experiment were significantly greater than the viscoelastic effects, indicating that the history-dependent changes in jejunal stiffness are more likely to reflect changes in the microelastic structures of the tissue than alterations in the viscous elements. Experimental studies involving bag distension in the gastrointestinal tract in which loading conditions are altered commonly fail to take these effects into account. Until now only few studies have been published on preconditioning effects and strain softening in the gastrointestinal tract [30-32].

Since strain softening in rubber materials is associated with "structural changes", one may think of it as damaging the tissue. However, strain softening may be a beneficial response as an adaptive, or restructuring, mechanism to an increased load in order to avoid damage to the tissue. The idea of such a function seems especially plausible in the gastrointestinal tract, where large dimensional changes occur in normal conditions. Thus, peristaltic bolus transport can stretch the intestinal wall in the vicinity of the bolus at low pressure, and strain softening may therefore have physiological relevance during normal bolus transport, as suggested by the low pressure range for strain softening. The time course of bolus mechanics and altered stiffness need more study.

Strain softening may also serve as a protective mechanism to reduce stresses during repeatedly high stretching. The data indicate the importance of strain softening at large increases in volume. High intraluminal pressures and dilatation are common in certain disease states associated with partial mechanical obstruction, which can occur in any part of the gastrointestinal tract. A maintained or repeated stretch of a segment of an organ rostral to the site of partial obstruction occurs because of abnormally high intra luminal pressures, reflecting both increased flow resistance and repetitive high amplitude contractions rostral to the obstruction site. The overstretching caused by the high pressures rostral to the obstruction may reduce the wall stiffness through strain softening mechanisms.

2.6. LAYERED MODELS

In recent years there has been a strong trend in research to pursue the idea that physical stress and strain are important factors in cell, tissue and organ physiology and in the pathogenesis of disease. The rationale is that the structure of any tissue is related to the function of that tissue, and the structure critically influenced by the physical strains to which it is subjected. These strains are related to stresses through constitutive equations.

The gastrointestinal tract is not a homogeneous tube. It is a composite, a multilayered tube with different physical properties in each layer of the wall and in each direction, the property of anisotropy as outlined in chapter 1. Mechanical data from individual layers add another dimension or characteristic in the hierarchy of the wall structure. To understand the mechanical function of the parts of the tract, it is necessary to know how stress and strain in the wall can be computed and how to determine the stress-strain relationships of the wall material. In most organs, it is impossible to separate layers without damaging the tissue. Gregersen *et al.* have described different mechanical properties in different layers of the esophagus, the only part of the gut where the mucosa is separable from the main muscle coat without apparently severe damage to the two layers. This high degree of separability comes from the relatively thick and loose submucosa in that organ as compared to the other parts of the gastrointestinal tract. The wall is dissected into two layers. One layer, the muscle layer, constitutes the main muscle coat consisting of the longitudinal and circular muscle layers, while the mucosa-submucosa layer contains most of the thickness of the submucosa, the thick muscularis of the mucosa, the lamina propria (a thin layer of connective tissue) and the squamous epithelium. The studies clearly show a difference in the opening angle and residual strains between the two layers. Fig. (**13**) shows a one-layer and a two-layer model of the no-load and zero-stress states. The residual strain curves are discontinuous at the interface between the mucosa-submucosa and muscle layers. This is a clear indication of shear forces acting at this interface. It has also been found that the circumferential incremental elastic modulus is a factor 7 higher in the mucosa-submucosa layer than in the muscle layer, whereas there is no difference in stiffness between the two layers in the longitudinal direction. These results show that the esophagus is a composite anisotropic structure.

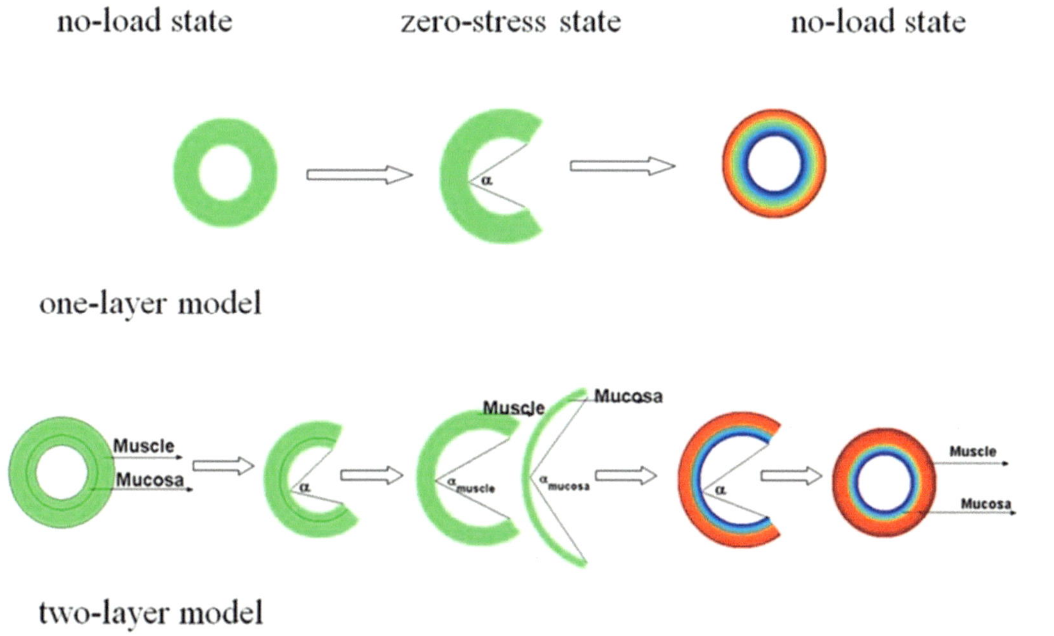

Figure 13: Schematics of the no-load and zero-stress states of one- and two-layered models. The figure shows that a two-layered organ needs to have its layers separated before the zero-stress state is obtained. If the zero-stress state is an open sector as shown in the figure, the mucosa will be compressed and the muscle stretched in the no-load state. [Courtesy of Professor Liao Donghua].

2.7. FLUID MECHANICS

Though flow is the result, the main consequence, of the motion of the gastrointestinal tract it is not the intention of this book to provide a detailed analysis of gastrointestinal fluid mechanics. The reason for this presumed lack is the relatively few data and valid models available for gastrointestinal flow. The gastrointestinal tract has received very little study from a fluid mechanical perspective. Furthermore, the matters are complicated due to the fact that the geometry of the tract is complex and the fluids are non-Newtonian (a viscous fluid for which the shear stress is linearly proportional to the rate of deformation). Water and air can be treated as nonviscous in many engineering problems but in relation to gastrointestinal function they probably cannot be regarded as nonviscous.

This chapter merely wishes to emphasize the most important concepts for the study of fluids in motion. Three significant fluid flow concepts are the following principles:

- conservation of mass,
- kinetic energy,
- momentum,

The equations of continuity, flow equations and equations evaluating dynamic forces exerted by flowing fluids are developed from these principles.

Gastrointestinal fluid mechanics are important in many processes. One important aspect is the gross mass transport of contents from the proximal to the distal tract. This gross transport is relatively easy to measure but its components are not. Secondary and retrograde flows, volume addition by secretion, volume reduction by absorption, physical changes in the fluid during flow, mixing of heterogeneous fluids, and gas production by microorganisms produce a complex flow system challenging even the most advanced contemporary fluid mechanical methods. However, fluid analysis is necessary to those who wish to truly understand gastrointestinal physiology. Ignoring gastrointestinal flow is just as ignorant as ignoring blood flow in the cardiovascular system.

Work on gastrointestinal flow seems much more scattered than work on visceral muscle contractility. This may be due to the difficulties involved in its study and the geometric complexity, the complex composition and properties of the fluids, and the flow types that seem to occur. Several studies have been published on gastrointestinal flow and the consequences of various types of contractions. Bioengineering principles were applied by Brasseur and coworkers in their work on bolus flow in the esophagus (see for example [12, 33]. The interested reader should consult the work by Bertuzzi [34], Denli, Stavitsky, Macagno, Fung, Tözeren, and Miftakhov (some references are given in the literature list). Though the complexity is enormous *in vivo*, fluid flow can to some extent be controlled in experimental set-ups *in vitro*. For example, it is possible to impose predetermined shear stresses to cultured cells in order to study their responses.

Flow and bolus transport in distensible organs like the gastrointestinal tract are influenced by many factors. The driving forces are the pressure generated by the contractile peristaltic events. To a much lesser extent, the hydrostatic force of gravity may have some importance. Biomechanical models show that determinants of flow include factors as the shape and size of the luminal cross-section, the size and viscosity of the bolus, and viscoelastic properties such as the elastic modulus, strain rate and shear properties of the wall. Luminal contents likely stretch the gastrointestinal wall, as least under some conditions where the contents propelled in front of a peristaltic contraction may distend the wall. This is the source of the idea that intestinal reflexes initiated by local stretch are important for generation of antegrade flow. Although it is debatable how much such reflexes actually regulate gastrointestinal flow in normal conditions, distension studies might help us to understand basic components for the complex fluid mechanical behavior.

Brasseur *et al.* studied esophageal flow properties, while primarily Macagno *et al.* described gastric emptying, antroduodenal mechanics, and intestinal flow properties. The literature on flow properties in the gastrointestinal tract was reviewed by Weems [35]. Stavitsky *et al.* used mathematical modeling to describe peristaltic transport in distensible tubes. The peristaltic transport modeling is based on the premise that the interaction between gastrointestinal elasticity and bolus transport can be understood by examining the fluid dynamics equations and equations describing gastrointestinal deformation.

2.8. APPENDIX

2.8.1. Some Notes on Commonly Used Mechanical Parameters

Many estimates of gastrointestinal stiffness are simplistic and unsound due to neglect of well-defined and fundamental characteristics as anisotropy, finite deformation, non-linear behavior, and viscoelasticity. Mechanics of the wall is so complex that even techniques with far better resolution than those currently available will not allow complete characterization of the three-dimensional gastrointestinal mechanical behavior *in vivo*. However, an ideal characterization is not always required. A general and valid means to express overall stiffness is necessary and useful. The following sections define and discuss commonly used elasticity parameters such as compliance and cross-sectional area distensibility.

2.8.1.1. Compliance

Compliance is a simple parameter defined as the change in luminal dimension (volume or cross-sectional area) divided by the corresponding change in pressure

$$C = \frac{\Delta V}{\Delta P}, \text{ or } C = \frac{\Delta CSA}{\Delta P} \qquad (2.39)$$

where C is compliance and V, CSA and P are volume, cross-sectional area, and pressure, respectively. Compliance is reciprocal to stiffness. Usually, it is provided as a single averaged value assuming it is linear. However, the compliance parameter merely expresses the differences in luminal dimensions between different pressures. Hence, the compliance parameter does not consider the actual degree of stretch occurring during luminal pressure loading, not does the parameter consider the variations in the unstressed basal luminal diameter, or in the wall thickness. As a result, compliance as an index of wall stiffness has virtually no validity in terms of the mechanics of the gut wall. Erroneous conclusions have often been drawn from gastrointestinal studies using compliance a mechanical parameter (see [16, 17] for details).

2.8.1.2. Cross-Sectional Area Distensibility

Volume of a distending bag as representative of a measure of cross-sectional area or diameter in a cylindrical viscus is invalid because the volume also may distribute towards the ends of the bag and elongate it. Therefore, in volume measurements it is necessary to know the distribution of the volume. However, direct methods to measure cross-sectional areas and circumferences exist. It is advantageous to express the distensibility in terms of cross-sectional area and transmural pressure rather than compliance. The distensibility is defined as the ratio of change of cross-sectional area (CSA) to the change in transmural pressure (P_{tm})

$$D = \left(\frac{1}{CSA_0}\frac{\Delta CSA}{\Delta P_{tm}}\right) \qquad (2.40)$$

where CSA_0 is the cross-sectional area at reference conditions. The distensibility parameter can be computed from a P-CSA curve. However, it may be useful to convert D into an incremental Young's modulus for distensions of the whole intestinal wall, modeled as a uniform cylinder with homogenous, isotropic walls. Use of an incremental Young's modulus is necessary due to the non-linearity between circumferential stress and cross-sectional area. A single elastic parameter can be defined by considering small departures from a mean, prestressed *in vivo* state and then linearizing the stress-strain curves. This is useful when the amplitude of the pressure is small. For pressure increase within a thin-walled isotropic gastrointestinal segment with constant length, Young's modulus E is related to the distensibility D by:

$$D^{-1} = \frac{\mathrm{E}}{1-\alpha^2}\frac{h}{d} \tag{2.41}$$

In this equation h is the wall thickness, d is intestinal diameter and α is Poisson's ratio (equal to 0.5 for incompressible materials).

2.8.1.3. Measurements and Analysis of Diameter Data

Gastrointestinal diameters can be obtained in several ways. For example *in vivo* diameters can be obtained by diagnostic imaging techniques. In mechanical terms diameter data need to be supported by pressure or force data. The pressure-diameter relation is popular among cardiovascular physiologists because pressure and diameter are important for flow and because diameters are measurable with ultrasound. The pressure-diameter relation is also useful for understanding gastrointestinal function. The compliance, expressed by the percentage change of diameter *versus* the change in transmural pressure, is a function of the of the intestinal wall thickness-to-diameter ratio and of the Young's modulus. On the assumption of thin-walled tube a simple estimation can be made. The tensile wall stress of a tube of diameter D is according to Laplace's formula given by

$$\tau_\theta = \Delta P_{tm}\frac{D}{2h} \tag{2.42}$$

where h is the wall thickness. The strain $\frac{\tau_\theta}{\mathrm{E}}$, which is also the change of diameter divided by the diameter, can be expressed as

$$\frac{\Delta D}{Do} = \frac{D}{2h\text{E}} \Delta \text{P}_{\text{tm}} \tag{2.43}$$

Consequently, the compliance $\frac{D}{2hE}$ is proportional to the diameter-wall thickness ratio, $\frac{D}{h}$, and inversely proportional to the material constant E.

The reference diameter D_0 can often not be determined at zero-pressure since the cross-sectional area of the intestine is not circular at zero pressure. The intestine becomes circular upon luminal pressure loading. Hence, it is useful to analyze the circularity of the cross-section as the pressure increases. The complex equations for a cylindrical shell can be simplified somewhat if the deformation is taken to be the same along each generator line. It is based on the following assumptions:

- the wall thickness-to-diameter ratio is small
- the material is isotropic and obeys Hooke's law with a Young's modulus E and Poisson's ratio ν
- an the no-load condition the cylinder has an elliptical cross-section so that its curvature can be expressed by the equation

$$\text{C}_0 = \frac{1}{a} + \frac{\varepsilon}{a} \cos 2\theta \tag{2.44}$$

In this equation a is the mean initial radius, θ is the polar angle, and ε is a measure of the cross-section ellipticity.

If the initial ellipticity is small (ε<<1), a simple solution can be analytically determined. It can be expressed as the change of curvature ΔC

$$\Delta \text{C} = \frac{-\frac{\varepsilon}{a}\cos 2\theta}{1 + \frac{Eh^3}{3(1-\upsilon^2)a^3\,\Delta P_{tm}}} \tag{2.45}$$

It demonstrates that when the transmural pressure $\Delta \text{P}_{\text{tm}}$ is zero, the denominator tends to infinity and ΔC = 0. Hence, the original elliptical cross-section is obtained. The solution becomes the following when the transmural pressure tends to infinity

$$\Delta C = \frac{-\varepsilon}{a}\cos 2\theta \tag{2.46}$$

This implies circular cross-section.

The transmural pressure at which the ellipticity is reduced to 5% of its initial value is accessible by letting the denominator of the fraction on the right hand side of Eq. 45 be 1.05

$$\Delta P_{tm} = \frac{E}{0.15\,(1-\upsilon^2)}\left(\frac{h}{a}\right)^3 \tag{2.47}$$

Consequently, assuming an incompressible material with $\nu = 0.5$, the transmural pressure required to reduce the ellipticity to 5% of the initial value can be computed given the material's Young modulus and thickness-to-radius ratio.

Parts of this chapter have been previously published in Complex Anorectal Disorders, 2005, pp. 72-104; in Basic and New Aspects of Gastrointestinal Ultrasonography, pp. 23-74; in Neurogastroenterology and Motility, volume 8, issue 4, pages 277-297, 1996; and in Biomechanics of the Gastrointestinal Tract. Springer Verlag 2002.

REFERENCES

[1] Nothnagel H. Zur chemischen reizung der glatten muskeln, zugleich als beitrag zur physiologie des darms. Arch Pathol Anat Physiol Klin Med 1882; 88: 1-11.

[2] Mall F. A study of the intestinal contraction. John Hopkins Hosp Rep 1896; 1: 37-75.

[3] Bayliss WM & Starling EH. The movements and innervation of the small intestine. J Physiol 1899; 24: 99-143.

[4] Bayliss VM & Starling EH. The movements and innervation of the small intestine. J Physiol 1901; 26: 125-138.

[5] Cannon WB. The mechanical factors of digestion. London: Edward Arnold 1911.

[6] Trendelenburg P. Physiologische and pharmacologische versuche über die dünndarmsperistaltik. Naunyn Schmiedeberg Arch Exp Pathol Pharmacol 1917; 81: 55-129.

[7] Fung YC. Biomechanics. mechanical properties of living tissues. 2nd edition. New York, Springer-Verlag 1993.

[8] Metry S, Arhan P, Chauvet G. A mathematical analysis of intestinal peristaltic waves. Med Eng Phys 1995; 17: 204-14.

[9] Srivastava LM, Srivastava VP, Sinha SN. Peristaltic transport of a physiological fluid. Part I. Flow in non-uniform geometry. Biorheology 1986; 20: 153-66.

[10] Tözeren A, Özkaya N, Tözeren H. Flow of particles along a deformable tube. J Biomechanics 1982; 15: 517-27.

[11] Macagno EO, Christensen J. Fluid mechanics of gastrointestinal flow. In: Johnson LR, Barret KE, Gishan FK, Merchant JL, Said HM, Wood JD. Eds. Physiology of the Gastrointestinal Tract. New York: Raven Press 1981; Chapter 10.
[12] Brasseur JG. Mechanical studies of the esophageal function. Dysphagia 1993; 8: 384-6.
[13] Miller LS, Vegesna AK, Brasseur JG, Braverman AS, Ruggieri MR. The esophagogastric junction. Ann N Y Acad Sci 2011;1232: 323-30.
[14] Li M, Brasseur JG. Non-steady peristaltic transport in finite-length tubes. J Fluid Mechanics 1993; 248: 129-51.
[15] Miftakhov RN, Abdusheva GR, Christensen J. Numerical simulation of motility patterns of the small bowel. part i-formulation of a mathematical model. J Theoretical Biology 1999; 197: 89-112.
[16] Gregersen H. Biomechanics of the gastrointestinal tract. Springer Verlag 2002.
[17] Gregersen H, Kassab GS. Biomechanics of the gastrointestinal tracT. J Neurogastroenterology Motil 1996; 8: 277-97.
[18] Liao D, Gregersen H, Hausken T, Gilja OH, Mundt M, Kassab GS. Analysis of surface geometry of the human stomach using real-time 3D ultrasonography *in vivo*. J Neurogastroenterology Motil 2004; 16: 315-324.
[19] Liao D, Zhao J, Fan Y, Gregersen H. Two-layered quasi-3D finite element model of the oesophagus. Med Eng Phys. 2004; 26: 535-543.
[20] Liao D, Wang P, Zhao J, Gregersen H. Validation of shape context based image registration method using digital image correlation measurement on a rat stomach. J Comp Med 2014; Article ID 504656, 7 pages.
[21] Frøkjær JB, Liao D, Bergmann A, *et al.* Three-dimensional biomechanical properties of the human rectum evaluated with magnetic resonance imaging. Neurogastroenterology Motil 2005; 17: 531-40
[22] Do Carmo, MP. Differential geometry of curves and surfaces. Englewood cliffs, NJ 1976.
[23] Regen DM. Tensions and stresses of ellipsoidal chambers. Ann Biomed Eng 1996; 24: 400-17.
[24] Fung YC. A first course in continuum mechanics. Englewood Cliffs: Prentice Hall. 1994.
[25] Chisena R, Zhao J, Gregersen H, Brasseur JG. Abstract WBC 2014
[26] Nash W. Theory and problems of strength. Third edition. USA. McGraw-Hill
[27] Dobrin PB. Mechanical properties of arteries. Physiol Rev 1978; 58; 397-460.
[28] Johnson M, Beatty M. The Mullins effect in uniaxial extension and its influence on the traverse vibration of a rubber string. Continuum Mech Thermodyn 1993; 5: 83-115.
[29] Emery JL, Omens JH, McCulloch AD. Strain softening in rat left ventricular myocardium. J Biomech Eng 1997; 119: 6-12.
[30] Gregersen H, Emery J, McCulloch AD. History-dependent mechanical behavior of the guinea-pig small intestine. Annals Biomed Eng 1998; 26: 1-9.
[31] Gao C, Petersen P, Liu W, Arendt-Nielsen L, Drewes AM, Gregersen H. Sensory-motor responses to volume-controlled duodenal distension. Neurogastroenterol Motil 2002; 14: 365-74.
[32] Pedersen J, Gao C, Egekvist H, *et al.* Pain and biomechanical responses to distention of the duodenum in patients with systemic sclerosis. Gastroenterology 2003; 124: 1230-39.
[33] Brasseur JG. A fluid mechanical perspective on esophageal bolus transport. Dysphagia 1987; 2: 32-9.
[34] Bertuzzi A, Salinari S, Mancinelli R, Pescatori M. Peristaltic transport of a solid bolus. J Biomechanics 1983; 16: 459-464.
[35] Weems WA. Intestinal fluid flow: Its production and control. In: Johnson LR, Christensen J, Jackson MJ, Jacobson ED, Walsh JH, Eds. Physiology of the gastrointestinal tract. New York, Raven Press 1987; Chapter 17, pp. 1-593.

CHAPTER 3

Methods in the Study of Gastrointestinal Mechanics

Abstract: Improved understanding of gastrointestinal function depends on improved study methods, for one can consider only those phenomena one can see the evidence for. New multidisciplinary efforts that include the use of bioengineering principles can overcome the problems imposed by the inaccessibility of the gut and by its complexity. This chapter outlines several bioengineering models, methods and analyses from studies of gastrointestinal mechanics. The three main themes are conventional techniques for recording gastrointestinal motor operations, methods involving the stimulation of the gut by distending it, and imaging technologies.

Keywords: Bioengineering model, distension, esophagus, functional luminal imaging, impedance planimetry, large intestine, manometry, small intestine, stomach, ultrasonography.

3.1. INTRODUCTION

Walter B. Cannon's seminal book, "The Mechanical Factors of Digestion" appeared in 1911, more than 100 years ago [1]. One might expect such an original book to initiate a burst of research in gastrointestinal mechanics so that the knowledge base would be large today. Sadly, this is not the case. Methodological developments have been slow and fundamental concepts remain to be investigated. The understanding of "gastrointestinal mechanical" disease has, in some respects, scarcely changed from that of Cannon's time.

Improved understanding depends on improved methods, for one can consider only those phenomena one can see the evidence for. New multidisciplinary efforts that include the use of bioengineering principles can overcome the problems imposed by the inaccessibility of the gut and by its complexity. New methods (and new concepts) in solid and fluid mechanics remain to be applied to the gastrointestinal tract where they might do much to bring our understanding of this system and its diseases closer to the standards of the 21st century.

This chapter outlines several bioengineering models, methods and analyses from studies of gastrointestinal mechanics, some old and some new that have not been fully reported before. The three main themes of this presentation are

- conventional techniques for recording gastrointestinal motor operations

Hans Gregersen and James Christensen

- methods involving the stimulation of the gut by distending it
- imaging technologies

3.2. MODELS FOR THE STUDY OF GASTROINTESTINAL MUSCLE MECHANICS AND OTHER FUNCTIONS

Many different kinds of animal models exist for the examination of the mechanical behavior of gut muscle. These range from strips of muscle maintained for study in a "physiological" environment *in vitro* to animals, including man, in whom appropriate devices exist to allow the mechanics of intact organs to be studied under conditions as nearly normal as possible. The following sections describe some useful models for the study of undisturbed motility, the motor responses to excitation by sensory and pharmacological stimulation, and the biomechanical aspects of motor operations in the gut. This book only considers *in vivo* models, *i.e.* models to be used in humans and live animals. The reader is referred to other literature regarding *in vitro* models and methods such as isolated perfused or non-perfused gastrointestinal segments, isolated muscle strips, cell cultures, the use of serosal strain gauges, and uni-axial, bi-axial and tri-axial tests. Reference [2] provides insight into such methods with referral to other literature.

Various factors must be considered carefully in the selection of a valid and useful model. For example, for studies involving the mechanoreceptors that affect motor function, it is important to know as fully as possible their mechanical milieu, their location, their orientation and other circumstances both *in situ* and in the experimental settings. Previous studies have suggested that mechanoreceptors are located both in the submucosa and in the muscle layers, in some organs at least. Their restriction to one or another layer of the gastrointestinal wall may well vary from one location or one organ to another. Zero-stress state studies have taught us that an intramural strain gradient exists under physiological conditions from the mucosa to the serosa. Hence, the mechanoreceptors located in different layers are exposed to different strains and stresses both at rest and during movements. Mechanoreceptors from different locations in the wall may thus have different zero-settings and respond in different ways to the same stimuli because the magnitudes of tensile stresses and strain during distension and the magnitudes of compressive stresses and strain during muscle contraction depend on the location in the wall. This indicates that any study involving receptor kinematics should keep these receptors in a milieu, especially a physical environment, as close as possible to the usual, using the intact organ *in vivo* or, less desirably, *in vitro*. These considerations also apply to the chemical environment, of course, because organs and tissues studied *in vitro* must certainly be hypoxic, at least to some degree.

3.2.1. *In vivo* Animal Models

For most investigators, the practical goal in research in gastrointestinal mechanics is the improved clinical management of disordered function. Thus, it would be ideal to examine only the human gastrointestinal tract. Ethical considerations, of course, limit the possibilities although some techniques are applicable in human studies. The recourse to animal studies often involves the unavoidable limitation of the necessity for anesthetic drugs. Thus, techniques that involve the ideal setting, the study of the gut *in situ*, suffer serious limitations.

Investigators often wish to see the effects of sensory nerve excitation on the mechanical behavior of the gut. Responses to mechanical, thermal, chemical and electrical stimulation of sensory nerves can be evaluated in both animals and man. The activation of the sensory system in such experiments can be verified in animals by measuring the electrical activity in afferent nerves. In contrast, the detection of sensory nerve activation in man can often be established only by the report of pain (or lesser sensations), a purely subjective method of measurement in which objectivity can only be crudely approached. The popularity of the measurement of evoked electroencephalographic potentials from the skull belies the limitations of the methodology, its difficulties of quantitation and uncertainties about the meaning of particular signals. The same can be said of PET scanning in such usages.

Animals with electrodes and tension-sensitive strain gauges chronically implanted on the gut are widely used to study its motor behavior in non-anesthetized and ambulant animals. In addition, many studies have been done on the surgically modified gut *in situ*, with various operations to make intestinal loops, anastomoses and fistulas. The investigators must wait for the animal to recover postoperatively for days or weeks. Such animals cannot be said to be truly normal for some time, perhaps much longer than the investigator wishes to wait to begin the studies, and some of these operations can be said to create a situation of chronic ill-health, perhaps deterioration, in the animal. These generic and inescapable complications of such an experimental approach rarely get much attention, but they should always come to the minds of those who use the derived data in developing a theory of gastrointestinal motility.

Such models for the study of the gut *in situ* have found much use in the description of the motions of the gut wall and the control of those motions, but they have had little place in the examination of the elastic properties. The several reasons for this include especially the difficulty in obtaining complete relaxation of visceral muscle *in vivo*. Methodological limitations have been partly overcome by the advent of techniques based on impedance planimetry and noninvasive imaging.

3.3. THE STUDY OF FLOW IN HUMANS

3.3.1. Methods for Measurement of Flow of Luminal Contents along the Gut

Two parameters are usually used to determine the flow of luminal contents along the gut *in vivo*: the flow rate and the transit time. The flow rate measures the volume flow along the gut in units of ml min^{-1}, whereas the transit time measures the velocity of the aboral movement of a luminal bolus in units of cm min^{-1}. Both are gross measures that provide no details about localized flows.

For the measurement of both flow rate and transit time, inert and non-absorbable markers are required. There are markers for both liquids and solids. The measurement of gastric emptying is possible with the radiographic observation of the emptying of a contrast medium or of radiopaque indissoluble radiopaque pellets mixed with a meal, or by the evaluation (with a computer-assisted gamma camera) of the diminution of radioactivity in the gastric area after the administration of a radiolabeled meal. Radiation hazards and the fact that the studies can only be performed with certain kinds of meals limit the use of such radiographic methods.

The flow of luminal contents in the small intestine is usually measured with liquid markers, soluble substances that flow along the gut together with the liquid phase of the ingested meal or infused luminal contents. Several kinds of liquid markers are commonly used. They include dye markers such as phenol red, chemical markers such as polyethylene glycol, heavy metal cation chelates such as CrEDTA or CoEDTA, and soluble isotopes. They can be measured photometrically, nephelometrically, by atomic absorption spectrometry, and by isotopic methods. For the measurement of flow rate, the marker is continuously infused into the gut and samples are removed downstream at defined intervals in time. For transit time measurements, the marker is injected as a bolus and samples are taken distally at short intervals of time. The transit time can be defined by different criteria, such as:

- the time period between injection and the first appearance of the marker,

- the time period until the maximum concentration of the marker is found, and
- the time period until the marker recovered reaches the value of 50%.

These measurements of flow rate and transit time in the small intestine are invasive because catheters are necessary for the administration of the marker and for the sampling of luminal contents. Intubation of the gut is not necessary, however, when isotopes are administered with a meal and the radioactivity is measured with a gamma camera in the regions of interest, (for example, at the terminal ileum or cecum). With such scintigraphic measurements, profiles of gastric emptying and colonic filling can be obtained repeatedly, allowing the small bowel transit to be determined consequently by calculation of the sizes of the images.

Another non-invasive test can measure the mouth-to-cecum or the duodenum-to-cecum transit time. When a non-absorbable carbohydrate such as lactulose is given with a meal or injected through a catheter into the duodenum, it provides an abundant substrate for bacterial fermentation when it arrives in the cecum (where bacteria flourish, in contrast to the small intestine). This fermentation generates hydrogen (among other things). The gas diffuses quickly into the blood stream and is exhaled in the breath where an abrupt peak in its concentration (as determined by the periodic sampling of the breath for analysis with special detectors) can be taken to signal the time of arrival of the substrate in the cecum. This is used clinically as an index of the mouth-to-cecum or duodenum-to-cecum transit time. This test is most frequently used in clinical studies because it is non-invasive and free of any hazards posed by radiation.

Such methods provide global measures of flow. Information about localized flow, such as that related to individual contractions, cannot be obtained by such techniques. In the esophagus, however, some information about the properties of flow in relation to peristalsis can arise from the use of radiographic techniques, observing the motions of radiopaque fluids during swallowing and with the spontaneous occurrence of secondary peristalsis.

Other non-invasive methods to examine flow are beginning to be used. Ultrasonography is useful for the study of gastric emptying, antroduodenal motility and antral size. In addition, the movements of the luminal contents across the pylorus can be studied by duplex sonography, a technique that combines real-time scanning with Doppler technology, as promoted by Dr. Hausken and the ultrasonography group in Bergen, Norway [3]. Some problems arise from individual anatomic variations that may prevent visualization in a single plane. Furthermore, the images may be blurred by subcutaneous fat and bowel gas.

3.4. THE STUDY OF THE MECHANICS OF THE HUMAN GASTROINTESTINAL TRACT

The preceding section surveyed the several techniques that can be used in the intact human gut to investigate its mechanical performance in terms of the consequence of that operation, the flow of luminal fluids. This section will deal in detail with manometry and bag distension, the two most common techniques used in human studies of gastrointestinal mechanical function. The section will also deal with imaging methods such as ultrasonography and MRI. All these methods can provide information about the physical characteristics of the gastrointestinal tract. Other techniques, such as electromyography, that can only partly suggest the mechanics of the muscle, will not be described here. Table **1**. outlines the most important methods and some of their features. The next sections go more into details with the methods and technologies.

Table 1. List of methods applicable in human studies. The table outlines the most common usage of the technologies.

Parameter **Method**	**Measure con-tractility (non-stimulated)**	**Provocatory test/measure distensibility**	**Provide measures mechanical stress or strain**	**Main parameters**
Conventional manometry	yes	no	no	Various motility indices
High-resolution Manometry	yes	no	no	Various motility indices based on color contour graphs
Intraluminal impedance (impedancometry)	Only during fluid flow	no	no	Various flow measures
Barostat	no	To some extent	no	Pressure-volume, compliance
Impedance Planimetry	yes	yes	Strain and stress resultants and moments	Pressure cross-sectional area, tension-strain relations
Multimodal stimulation	yes	yes	Strain and stress resultants and moments	Pressure cross-sectional area, tension-strain relations, thermal index, acid index

Table 1: contd….

Functional luminal Imaging probe (FLIP)	yes	yes	Strain and stress resultants and moments	Pressure and serial cross-sectional area, tension-strain relations
Endoscopic ultrasonography	yes	Yes if combined with bag distension	Strain (stress if combined with pressure recordings	Strain, longitudinal extension
Ultrasonography (abdominal scanning)	often	Yes if combined with bag distension	Strain (stress if combined with pressure recordings)	2D-3D geometry that may be combined with pressure measurements. Strain rate imaging
Magnetic Resonance Imaging	To some extend	Yes if combined with bag distension	Strain (stress if combined with pressure recordings)	2D-3D geometry that may be combined with pressure measurements.

3.4.1. Manometry

Manometry is commonly used to record the mechanical activity of the gastrointestinal tract. It detects the changes in luminal pressure caused by contractions. Two methods exist for measurement of luminal pressure. In one, pressure-sensitive strain gauges are placed in the lumen of the gastrointestinal tract. The other involves the measurement of pressures from a small open-tipped low-compliance catheter that is perfused very slowly with water with a low-compliance pump; its tip is placed in the lumen to allow the measurement of pressure changes that result from contractions.

In the solid state technique, the strain-gauge sensor is placed on a probe in the lumen of the organ. Normally, several sensors are placed in tandem on the probe. The technique provides good dynamic characteristics, and it can be used in portable systems for long-term recordings. Its discrimination of contractions in space depends on the number and spacing of the sensors. Nowadays more than 30 electrodes may be used in high-resolution manometry (HRM).

The perfusion technique is still widely used but it is prone to more errors than the strain gauge technique. Its popularity reflects mainly its low cost. It has no other advantage, such as accuracy, better discrimination, or better patient acceptability. The dynamic characteristics, though poor by engineering standards, are sufficient to record intraluminal pressures in most parts of the gastrointestinal tract. Although the use of the perfusion technique and the solid state technique began about 4 decades ago, there has been very little fundamental improvement since it began, perhaps except for the new way of presenting the data as color contour plots which seems easier to interpret for the human brain.

Most probes have a diameter of less than 5 mm. When a lumen-occluding contraction occurs in the gastrointestinal tract, pressure increases in the vicinity of the side hole or solid state transducer. With the perfused system the obstruction of the flow through the hole out of the channel results in counter-pressure in the fluid in the channel, rising to the same pressure as the luminal pressure. The pressure in the fluid-filled channel is, of course, detected continuously by the transducer. The analogue signal from the transducer is amplified and on-line recordings are after analogue-to-digital conversion displayed on computer monitors.

A special case is presented in gastrointestinal sphincters where a maintained contraction of the circular layer of muscle occludes the lumen for much of the time. Here, the force of the tonic (maintained) contraction can be recorded with the perfusion technique in either of two ways. In the so-called "stationary" technique, the investigator pulls the probe until one of its catheter openings enters the sphincter (as shown by a sudden rise in the baseline pressure detected) and then stops there to observe the behavior of the sphincter over a period of time. In the other method, called the "pull-through" technique, the investigator pulls the probe slowly and continuously through the sphincter and observing the pressures in all the catheter channels as they move first into and then out of the sphincter.

These two techniques have different sources of error. In the stationary technique, the error arises from the fact that the pressure recorded within the sphincter differs with different positions of the catheter opening, and from the fact that the catheter may shift. Thus, one sampling point cannot be taken as representative of the whole muscle ring and one cannot be sure that the sampling point has not changed. The "pull-through" technique does not allow assessment of the time-dependence of sphincter contraction, which is known to be considerable.

These limitations can be partly overcome by the use of a catheter constructed with a short sleeve sealed over one side hole so that the pressure over the length of the sleeve is integrated. This is essentially a small non-distensible bag. This is occasionally still used clinically in the study of the lower esophageal sphincter where respiratory movements tend to move the probe forwards and backwards in relation to the sphincter.

It is important to recognize that the technique in non-sphincteric regions only measures occlusive phasic contractions from the circular muscle layer. Those contractions that do not reduce the lumen to the diameter of the tiny probe cannot be detected. This means that perfusion manometry displays only the most forceful events.

From the point of view of the engineer, such methods seem inadequate. It is true that the two manometric techniques, the perfused technique and the solid state technique, both record the same number of contractions in the canine duodenum, but both record only about 90% of the spontaneous and generated neurogenic contractions that are detected by strain gauges sewn on the serosa. Such strain gauges also fail to record movements of the intestinal wall seen with the naked eye in experiments with the intestine exposed. Even worse, perfusion techniques also record artifactual pressure peaks that are produced by somatic movements such as those associated with respiration.

Furthermore, when the propagation velocities of contractions are calculated from the time of appearance of two peaks at adjacent points on the intestine, two important facts are usually ignored because they cannot be assessed or controlled: First: the gut itself shortens a great deal in contractions; second, the soft and contracting organ commonly telescopes on the stiffer probe.

3.4.2. Distension Techniques

Distension of a bag placed in the gastrointestinal lumen is commonly done *in situ* to investigate the force-deformation relationship and the motor responses to mechanosensitive receptors. The distension of a viscus is also used in the investigation of non-cardiac chest pain, in the treatment of diseases such as atherosclerosis, in compressing bleeding esophageal varices caused by liver disease, and to forcefully open the lower esophageal sphincter in esophageal achalasia.

In research, but not in the clinic, distension of a viscus is often done *in vivo* and *in vitro* with simultaneous measurements of pressure, volume, and cross-sectional area. Furthermore, distension can be combined with imaging techniques as B-mode ultrasonography to obtain geometric data on the cross-section and wall thickness of a viscus when these are important data to get in a research investigation. Basic considerations regarding distension of a bag as a mechanical tool are provided below.

Distensions can be performed in several ways. When the pressure is controlled, the procedure follows an isobaric protocol. When the volume is controlled, it is named an isovolumetric protocol. The distension test can be done stepwise (or staircase-wise) by which each step increase is made in successive uniform increments, or randomly, by which new magnitudes of distension are imposed in no particular order. In contrast, a ramp-wise distension consists of the continuous inflation of the bag at a wide range of possible rates (Fig. **1**). Volume is easily controlled, whereas the control of bag pressure, diameter, cross-sectional area, tension and strain are more difficult and require special techniques. Though volume is easily controlled, it may not provide a uniform and reproducible stimulus of the wall (see later). Selection of a proper test protocol depends on the purpose of the study. At the outset, many considerations may have to be made, but the most important are:

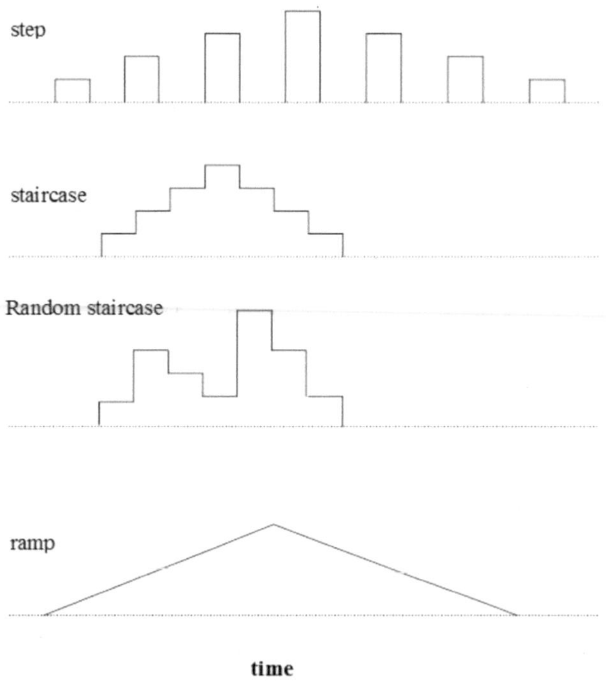

Figure 1: Examples of step, staircase and ramp testing schemes. The time scale is arbitrary. Normally the ramp test is by far the fastest to run because equilibrium is not required. The scheme does not take preconditioning into consideration.

- ***Reproducibility.*** This factor is often not considered in studies *in vivo*. In order to obtain reproducible results, the tissue must be preconditioned: That is, the test must be repeated until the responses become stable before data are actually collected. The investigators must decide on the criteria for stability from the initial experience. Fig. (**2**) shows an example of preconditioning behavior during repeated mechanical loadings.

- ***Loading Pattern.*** The duration of loading and the magnitude of loading are important for the definition of physiological processes in the tissue and for determining whether or not reversible or irreversible damage occurs. Stepwise distension, whether incremental or random, can be especially troublesome because it can impede blood flow to the distended part for considerable time periods. It is also important to know that this sort of distension is most suited to studies where the viscoelastic properties of the tissue are of interest, because, in step distension, the tissue is suddenly strained or stressed. Ramp distension, in contrast, provides a continuously increasing load where the time-dependent properties of the tissue do not come into play (see chapter 2 for more information on viscoelasticity).

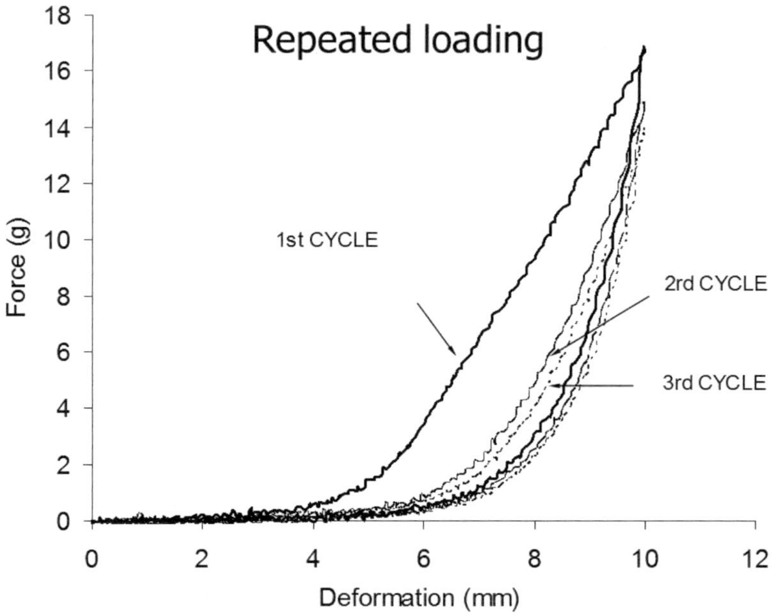

Figure 2: Two mechanical loadings of a gastrointestinal tissue tube. The first cycle shows a large hysteresis with huge difference between the loading and unloading curves. The second cycle shows a loading curve that is close to the unloading curve of the first cycle and the hysteresis is much less. The third cycle is not far away from that of cycle 2 but this tissue needed a fourth cycle (not shown) to be fully preconditioned. The data clearly demonstrates that it is important to precondition the tissue during testing (Modified from [2]).

3.4.2.1. Consideration of Geometric Factors in Distension Studies

Since most distensibility data from various gastrointestinal organs have been obtained mainly *in vivo* by bag distension methods, consideration to such an approach will be given in greater detail. The most important aspects relate to the

- probe design,
- experimental design,
- method of stimulation and measurement,
- geometry and mechanical properties of the bags,
- properties of the tissue and its surroundings (tethering to other organs)
- assumptions for the analysis.

The boundary of a geometrically measurable parameter must be in complete contact with the measurand; that is, in the process of measuring the cross-sectional area of a tube or the volume of an organ of any shape, the whole circumference and surface area of the bag should be in contact with the tissue. This ideal is never completely attained in volume measurements in the intestine and the stomach, of course. It is important to ensure that the applied pressure is properly transmitted to the tissue; that is, the bag must be large enough that it does not contribute its own elastic properties to the measurements. If this cannot be done, a correction must be made. In other words, the pressure of the distension must be transmitted entirely to the organ wall itself which, with a large enough bag, can be assumed so long as the surrounding structures do not interfere (for example, by tethering). Hysteresis of the bag and infusion system is usually negligible but it should always be looked for by testing. Friction between the viscus wall and the bag wall is in our experience not negligible. That is, the longitudinal strain in the wall depends on whether the segment is distended by a bag or by filling the lumen with fluid, even at comparable loads.

To avoid difficulties in the interpretation of results in studies involving the distension the intestine, the bag should be rather short in order to provide a localized distension to the size and approximate the shape of a bolus. In some studies (for example by Rouillon and Bell [4, 5], very long bags have been used. It has little physiological significance to distend the intestine with a long bag. Also, data on tone and distensibility may be difficult to interpret in such a case because reflex stimulation and inhibition of phasic activity will likely occur at the same time at the proximal and distal end of the bag time respectively with the result that the volume and pressure in the bag do not change much despite all the activity in the response. That is to say, the volume measured in a long bag may show little change even though the shape of the bag changes considerably. Conversely, great volume changes may accompany small shape changes. The results depend on the phasic contractility in the segment under study. This explains why the definition of specific tone (see Chapter 4) does not apply for barostat studies (a method for combined pressure-volume measurement) since this technique provides a three-dimensional measure of tone that is difficult to differentiate from phasic contractility. It may detect "tetanic tone", a summation of phasic contractions.

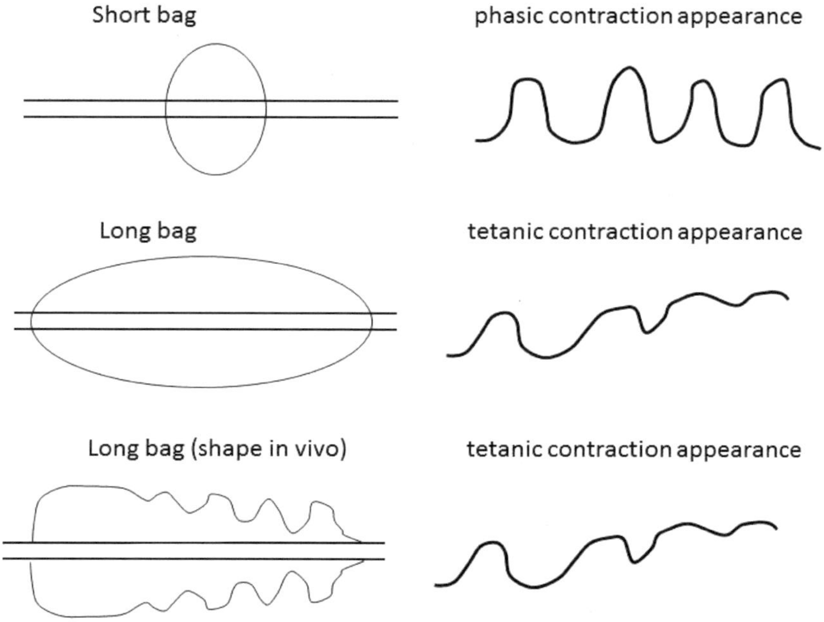

Figure 3: A schematic illustration of a commonly used bag type for esophageal and intestinal studies. A short bag is shown at the top including how the pressure tracings would look like at a constant volume. The two lower diagrams show a longer bag in a distended configuration and when distended *in vivo* with forces from contractions influencing its shape. The pressure tracing in the long bag will reflect a sum of the pressure acting along the length of the bag. Often several contractions may occur at the proximal end of the bag moving fluid to the distal end of the bag where the intestine is relaxed due to reflex mechanisms.

The dynamic characteristics of the measurement system also make it difficult to compare results from different studies. For example, short bags encounter only a few contractions while long bags sum up phasic contractions in a "tetanic tone" pattern (Fig. **3**). That is, large bags must integrate local events within their domain and these may be opposite in sense. Consequently, these limitations of bag techniques make it necessary that measurements be obtained at one location. Also, the luminal cross-sectional area must be measured rather than the volume. In any case, the bag must be short.

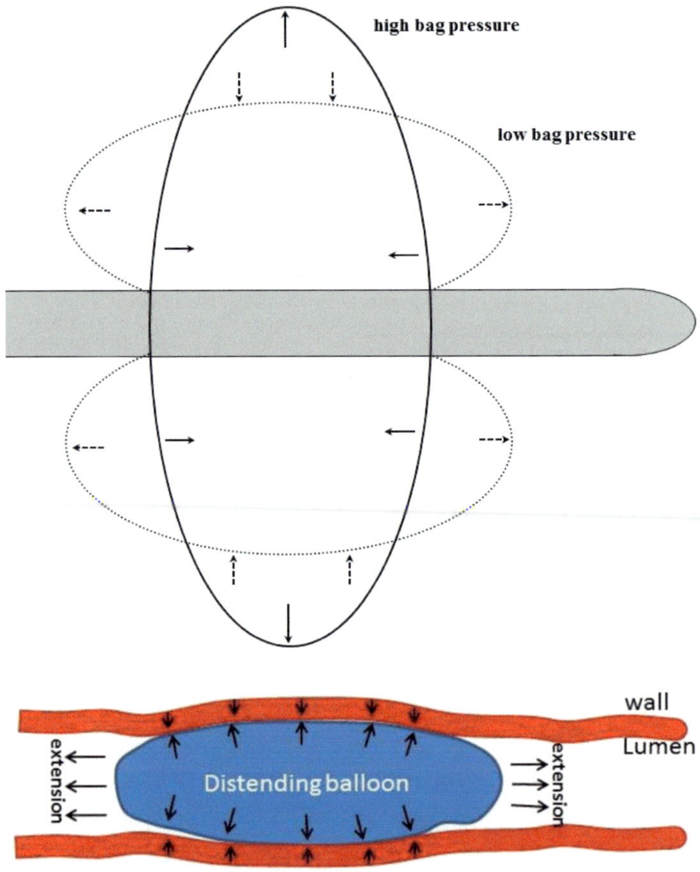

Figure 4: A schematic illustration of commonly used bag (balloon) types for esophageal and intestinal studies. In the top figure two degrees of distension is shown for a fairly rigid bag. The solid line shows when the pressure is high, resulting in a large diameter and an almost spherical bag geometry. The dotted line illustrates a lower pressure where the radial stretch is less. Due to the finite dimension of the bag, the bag will appear longer and bulge out in both ends. For this reason, volume measurements are not usable in calculations of cross-sectional distensibility, tension and strain. The arrows indicate the direction of forces for the bag pressurized with the lower pressure (dotted line arrows) and for the higher pressure (solid line arrows). In the bottom figure it is illustrated for a longer elastic balloon how it tends to expand in axial direction due to the resistance to deformation of the wall.

Another significant limitation is the fact that the bag will inescapably tend to elongate as it fills rather than to distend the organ wall by radial expansion alone because of the resistance to deformation of the viscus in the radial direction. (This must exceed the resistance of the viscus to extension in the direction of the axis of the cylinder because it is hollow). The magnitude of the elongation depends on the bag material and is most apparent with short bags, but it must occur to some degree with any bag (Fig. **4**).

This has several important implications:

- Parameters such as wall tension and compliance will be over-estimated.
- The large variation in intestinal size between subjects gives rise to a large variation in the pressure-volume relationship and compliance.
- Elongation will increase the stimulation area so that the receptive field for sensory receptors in the viscus wall field will be larger.
- Even a small error in the volume-to-diameter conversion in the low-pressure range, as shown in Fig. (**4**), will affect the results of a tension-strain analysis.

To overcome these invalidating problems, impedance planimetry and endo-sonographic methods for measurement of luminal cross-sectional area have been developed. Cross-sectional area as a function of pressure provides essential information on luminal dimensions during loading and, with further mechanical analysis, data on the material properties of the wall.

Biomechanical analysis depends on geometric factors and geometric assumptions must be made to simplify the analysis. For example, the Laplace equation is valid for a thin-walled circular tube or sphere. In more complex geometries, the mechanical models are more complex and require numerical analysis. This has obvious consequences for the interpretation of data on tone and distensibility. However, very few studies consider the proper geometry and estimate the degree to which the tubular sections of the gastrointestinal tract are circular or the degree to which the stomach is spherical.

Because of the serious limitations explained above, those bag distension techniques that are based wholly on simultaneous pressure-volume measurements will not be further considered in this book. The actual measurements of pressure and volume may be accurate. The derived parameters, such as tension, however, must be considered invalid because of the insupportable assumptions that must be made, the errors caused by the nearly universal failure to appreciate bag elongation, and the failure to detect the simultaneous and events that must occur within the domain of long bags.

The following is a description of impedance planimetry, a technique based on fewer assumptions and better validation using bioengineering principles than the pressure-volume methods.

3.4.2.2. Impedance Planimetry

Impedance planimetry is a technique for the measurement of luminal cross-sectional area (CSA) in hollow organs like cylindrical tubes. The term, impedance planimetry, as suggested in 1991 [6], defines a method to measure the size of a plane using measurement of electrical impedance. Impedance planimetry utilizes a simple electrical principle based on Ohm's law. However, as with any new technology, the static and dynamic properties of the system and the potential sources of error must be considered. The few sources of error in impedance planimetry can easily be controlled.

The history of impedance planimetry. About four decades ago, Harris and coworkers described a method using the principles of impedance measurements for the assessment of CSA in the ureter [7]. The measurement system consisted of four or more electrodes placed in a linear array on a thin probe to be passed into the ureter. If a voltage was applied to the two end electrodes, a current flowed between them when a urine bolus passed the electrodes. During the current flow, the investigators recorded the potential difference between the two detection electrodes, the other pair of electrodes located between the two end electrodes. Since an inverse relation exists between the potential difference in an enclosed volume of a conducting fluid and the CSA, the latter could be deduced from such measurements of potential differences. The system was made usable for measurements of CSA, contraction velocity and bolus shape in the ureter.

Apparently without knowing the paper by Harris and other papers following from other groups, Fisher and coworkers in 1978 applied a variant of the method for the determination of bolus velocity and clearance in the human esophagus using a multi-electrode system [8]. Fass and Silny repeated this work in a series of papers from 1990, again apparently in ignorance of the previous work [9].

Colstrup further developed the impedance method for further urological use in 1983 [10, 11]. He introduced a system with the electrodes placed inside a fluid-filled non-conductive latex bag (a balloon) for the measurement of compliance, defined as the change in cross-sectional area divided by the change in bag pressure. This system had the advantage that the flow of current was confined to the fluid in the bag. The system proved sufficient for extensive studies of the active and passive properties of the urethra wall in healthy females and in those with stress incontinence (Lose and Colstrup [12].

Gregersen introduced Colstrup's bag method for studies of the gastrointestinal tract in 1988 [13]. The relatively large size of the gastrointestinal tract demanded the further development of the measuring system. The modified system was named "impedance planimetry" in 1991, the term reflecting the measurement of a two-dimensional variable from the measurement of electrical impedance. Impedance planimetry has during the past decades been further developed into a tensiometer or tensiostat, a multimodal probe, and into a functional luminal imaging technology by Gregersen and coworkers (see later in this chapter).

The principle of cross-sectional area measurement. Consider a linear array of four electrodes mounted on a catheter (Fig. **5**), and consider Ohm's law. When a constant alternating current I is induced in an electrical volume conductor by the two outer (excitation) electrodes, the potential difference V between the two inner (detection) electrodes is

$$V = I\,Z \qquad (3.1)$$

If the two excitation electrodes are sufficiently far from the detection electrodes, a uniform electrical field is created in the vicinity of the detection electrodes. Z, the electrical impedance of the fluid, can also be expressed as $d\,\delta^{-1}\,CSA^{-1}$ with d as the distance between the detection electrodes and δ the conductivity of the fluid. Thus, the potential difference between the detection electrodes can be expressed as

$$V = I\,d\,\delta^{-1}\,CSA^{-1} \qquad (3.2)$$

I, d, and δ are constant within an experiment. The current I in the impedance planimetry systems used nowadays is often an AC current of 100 microamperes and the detection electrode distance is 1-2 mm. The conductivity of the fluid (usually diluted saline is used) is constant as long as the temperature is kept constant. Thus, V is inversely proportional to the CSA

$$V = k\,CSA^{-1} \qquad (3.3)$$

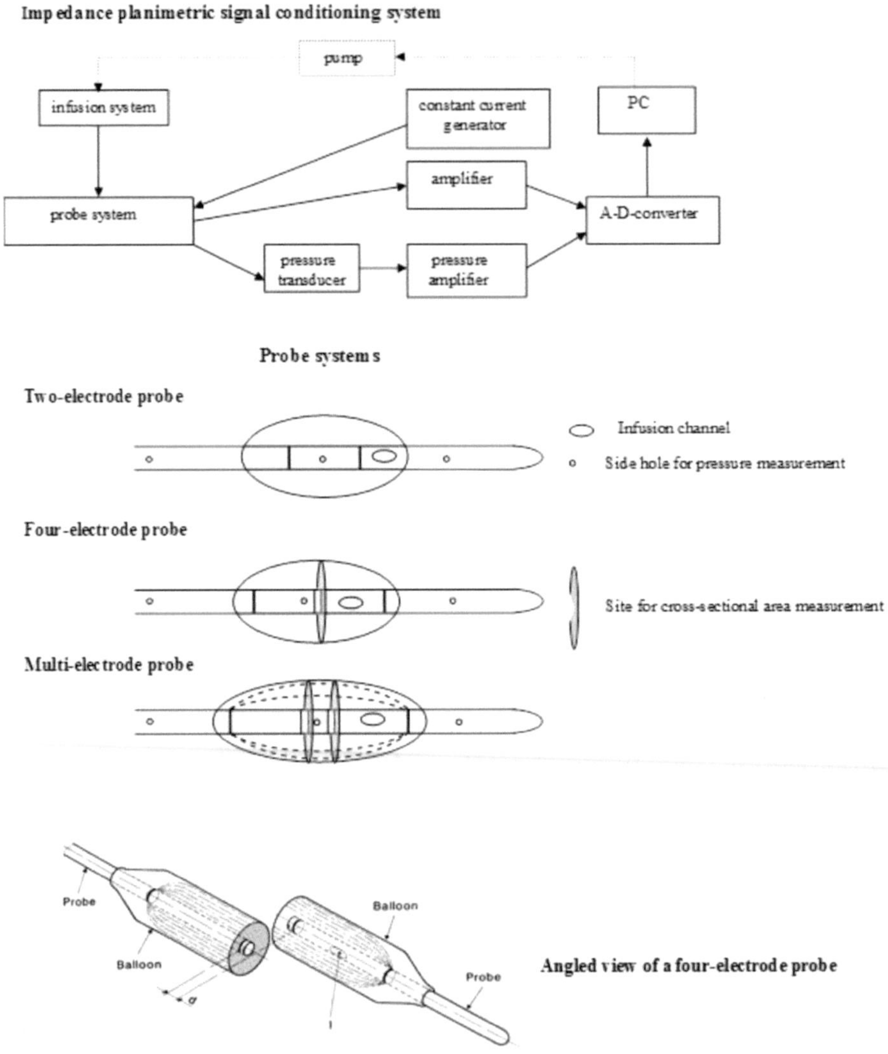

Figure 5: Schematics of the impedance planimetry and tensiostat system. Three different probe designs are illustrated (the four electrode system is shown from two angles). The system renders possible pressure-cross-sectional area measurements, evaluation of peristaltic reflex responses and standardization of the stimulation stimulus in terms of tension or strain. The group of dash lines (shown only inside the two bottom bags) forming a field between the two outer excitation electrodes represents the flow of constant AC current. In the tensiometer system a computer-controlled pump is added to the system as shown by the dotted lines. The computer calculates tension in real time from measurements of bag pressure and CSA and remote controls the pump to infuse/withdraw fluid from the bag in order to change tension. I and d in the bottom figure denote the infusion channel (shown by other symbols in the upper figures) and the distance between the detection electrodes.

Direct proportionality between the output V and the CSA can be obtained by means of reciprocating software. After reciprocation, Eq. 3.3 can be written as

$$V = k\,\text{CSA} \tag{3.4}$$

where k is a calibration constant.

The electrical field created by the current from the excitation electrodes is confined to the conducting fluid inside the bag that encompasses the electrodes on the probe, when such a bag is present. If the bag is not used, the current passes through the fluid in the lumen of the gastrointestinal tract (and, to a lesser degree, through its wall). The bag system has been very useful for distension studies. The pressure or volume inside the bag can be controlled either by raising or lowering a fluid container that is connected to the bag by a channel, or by a pump. The impedance system without using a bag is known as intraluminal impedance, despite the fact that the current is not confined to the lumen but also flows in the wall, or as impedancometry. This technology is being used to study bolus transport in the esophagus.

The four-electrode system can be extended to include many sets of detection electrodes (multi-electrode systems) so that serial cross-sections can be obtained along the longitudinal axis. This has the advantage that the three-dimensional geometry of the bag can be modeled, and the spatial and temporal distribution of contractions can be described in more detail. This system is now named functional luminal imaging probe or in brief FLIP.

The paper by Harris from 1971 on ureteral physiology still stands as one of the most important methodological papers [7]. Other papers also deal with possible sources of error in impedance planimetric measurements [11-13]. The errors can be divided into those errors directly associated with the CSA measurement and those errors related to the derived biomechanical parameters. Errors related to the CSA measurements cover changes in conductivity, temperature, dislocation of the probe from the center axis, and slope of the organ wall. The possible sources of error are described in detail in previous papers and are not a concern if the studies have been done carefully.

3.4.2.3. Techniques based on Impedance Planimetry

Tensiometer – tensiostat. The addition of a tensiometer and tensiostat for the measurement and control of circumferential wall tension and strain in the gastrointestinal tract have further developed impedance planimetry. This development was prompted by the need for better control of the distension stimulus, since the mechanoreceptors in the intrinsic and extrinsic pathways respond to changes in stress and strain rather than to changes in pressure or volume. The main assumptions on which this technique is based are that

- Both pressure and CSA are reliably measured,
- the use of Laplace's law is valid, and
- the dynamics of the stimulation and recording system are adjusted to the organ under study.

A diagram of the mechanical arrangement for the tensiometer is outlined in Fig. (**5**). The system consists of a probe with four ring electrodes and a 4-cm-long and 5-cm-diameter bag, an impedance planimeter, pressure transducer, pressure amplifiers, and a pump with an interface to a PC with dedicated software. The pump, remotely controlled by a PC, infuses and withdraws fluid from a reservoir into the bag mounted on a multi-lumen 14F probe. The pressure is measured inside the bag using a low-compliance perfused pneumohydraulic system connected to the external transducer. With this system, the bag pressure and CSA are measured by means of manometry and impedance planimetry, and the signals are amplified, analogue-to-digital converted and transferred to the computer for real-time display and tension computation. The pump is not used in *open-loop feedback mode* (tension measurement mode, pressure or volume control mode). Hence, the system records variations in tension when the bag is inflated to a given pressure, volume or CSA. In *closed-loop feedback mode* (tension control mode), the PC regulates the pump to infuse and withdraw fluid to obtain the selected tension. The infusion rate of the pump is regulated by a software subroutine.

The system has been validated *in vitro* by using various sized PVC tubes and pressure test chambers. Furthermore, instant changes in pressure and CSA were imposed to test how the system reacts in tension measurement mode and tension control mode. The tension error is a function of pressure and radius. Error propagation analysis showed, in the pressure and radius ranges from 10-100 mmHg and 5-20 mm, that the tension error was 1.1-5.6%. The tension resolution was approximately 0.1 mm mmHg. The paper by Gregersen, Barlow and Thompson from 1999 gives further details and physiological data [14].

Multimodal stimulation. It is obvious that the reaction to a single stimulus of a given modality can represent only a limited fraction of the entire pain experience since pain is a multidimensional perception. Combining different methods for stimulation and assessment of perceptions will imitate the clinical situation where many nerves and pathways are activated. Hence, the method will give a more comprehensive and differentiated information about the nociceptive system compared to stimuli using single or a few modalities. For comprehensive experimental studies mimicking the clinical situation, a multimodal testing approach must be used where the test battery will increase the probability for activation of a range of relevant nervous mechanisms. Such sophisticated methods will be able to select the best test procedures to explore different basic aspects of pain as well as pharmacological modulations. Especially if the stimulation includes modalities known to evoke peripheral as well as central sensitization, the likelihood that a model will mimic clinical pain is high despite the non-harmful nature of the stimulation [15]. In the gastrointestinal tract, difficulties with access to the organs and technical limitations of the currently models have made the multimodal stimulation approach difficult. Some authors such as Accarino have combined mechanical and electrical stimuli [16] or mechanical and chemical stimuli [17]. In a study by Sarkan in the esophagus mechanical and electrical stimuli were combined with sensitization to acid [18]. Drewes and Gregersen developed a multimodal model with combined mechanical, electrical, cold and warmth stimuli of the esophagus together with acid sensitisation [15] (Figs. **6** and **7**).

The multimodal approach gives the possibility for a differentiated stimulation of receptors in the superficial and deep layers of the gut. The induction of hyperalgesia with, for example, acid perfusion and for evoking central phenomena such as summation, allodynia and referred pain makes the model clinically relevant with respect to increase the knowledge of peripheral and central pain mechanisms [19-21]. The pain assessment should ideally also be multimodal and for example include quantitative and qualitative sensation, assessment of referred pain and neurophysiological measurements.

Multimodal studies done in the human esophagus demonstrate that the procedure can be done safely, if proper security devices are built into the equipment and testing scheme. All modalities can induce pain separately and in combination. A stimulus such as acid infusion in the esophagus changes the sensitivity to mechanical stimulation, indicating the polymodal nature of at least some receptor populations.

Furthermore, central phenomena such as temporal summation and viscero-somatic relations can be studied. This mimics the mechanisms that appear to be active in clinical diseases of the gastrointestinal tract. Pharmacological modulation of the output variables is a potent option that should be tested in the future

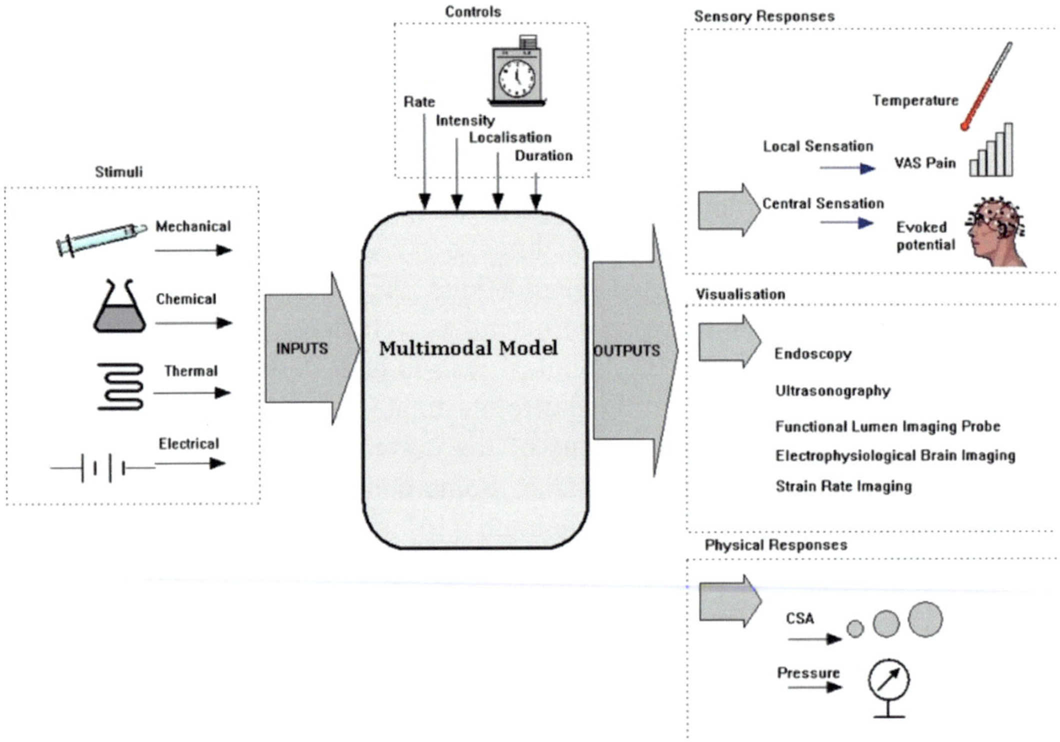

Figure 6: Sketch of advanced multimodal system with mechanical, chemical, thermal and electrical stimulations (input), controls, and output in terms of sensory and physical responses and imaging outcomes. Courtesy of Dr. Asbjørn Drewes.

Chronic pain is characterized by modifications of the central nervous system such as central sensitization. Hence, decreased thresholds to normal stimuli such as stools and air in the gastrointestinal tract may contribute to many of the symptoms reported by patients with inflammatory and functional diseases in the gut. Phenomena relating to sensitization of the CNS are enhanced responses to repeated stimulation, allodynia/hyperalgesia and increase in the referred pain area [15]. Central mechanisms are important in functional gut disorders. Chemical stimulation may evoke sensitization, for example, an increased response to mechanical, electrical and thermal stimuli after chemical sensitization have been demonstrated [15, 18].

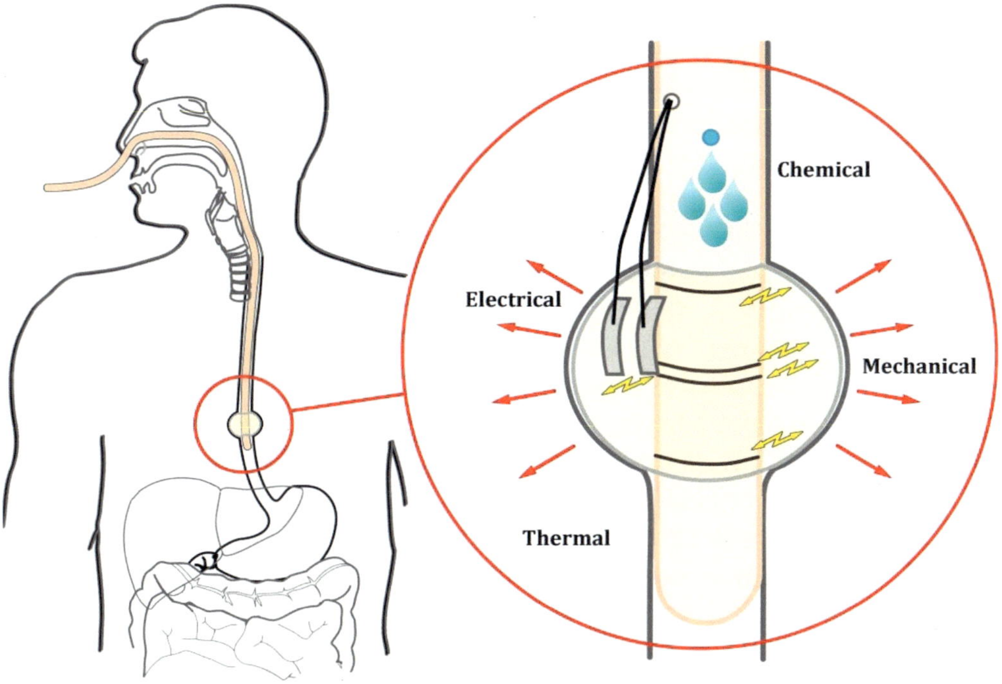

Figure 7: Multimodal probe.

Advanced muscle studies in humans. Geometric parameters such as the length and the luminal diameter, and the passive and active properties of tissues are important for the transport function of the gastrointestinal tract as well as for the sensory properties. Tools have been developed for studying both the active (phasic and tonic contractions) and passive behavior of the gut using impedance planimetric distension before and during administration of inhibitory drugs [15, 22, 23]. Tension, stress and strain are of principal interest because these parameters give information about the elastic properties, and mechanoreceptors respond more directly to these parameters than to pressure and volume. Furthermore, the muscle function is better evaluated when the forces and tensions themselves can be measured as compared to the pressures generated by contractions. New techniques to study gastrointestinal muscle function have been developed recently. For example, ramp-controlled distension in the human esophagus before and during administration of butylscopolamine allows the differentiation between passive, tonic and phasic-tonic tensions. The tensions are plotted as function of the luminal radius to reveal an *in vivo* tension-strain diagram, an analysis somewhat similar to the isometric length-tension curves obtained in muscle strips *in vitro*. The active tension-radius curve analyses how the initial length changes of a muscle affect the ability of the muscle to develop force (tension).

In addition, the change in tension during individual distension-induced contractions (afterload) as function of the radius immediately before the contractions (preload radius) can be analyzed. Similarly the change in radius during distension-induced contractions can be plotted as function of the preload radius. These diagrams correspond to heart function curves in terms of the ventricular stroke work as function of the mean atrial pressure. Such curves are similar to the well-known Frank-Starling mechanism in the heart [24]. The Frank-Starling mechanism can be explained the following way. When an extra amount of blood flows into the ventricles, the cardiac muscle itself is stretched to greater length. This causes the muscle to contract with increased force because the myosin and actin filaments are brought to a more nearly optimal degree of interdigitation for force generation. The importance of the concept of preload and afterload in cardiac physiology is that in many abnormal functional states of the heart and circulation, the pressure during filling of the ventricle or the arterial pressure against which the ventricle must contract, or both, are severely altered from the normal. This concept may be useful for the evaluation of normal esophageal physiology in aging and in the pathophysiology of gastro-esophageal reflux disease, systemic sclerosis, obstruction, achalasia, functional chest pain, spasms and other esophageal disorders.

Examples of *in vivo* length-tension diagrams, preload-afterload diagrams and force-velocity data are given in Fig. (**8**) and the reader is referred to papers by Pedersen, Zhao and Liao [25-27].

Functional luminal imaging. Gastrointestinal sphincters are narrow zones along the gastrointestinal tract that divide it into compartments and control flow of gases, liquids and solids. These regions contain tonically contracted muscle rings to maintain a barrier and to act as a valve between hollow organ segments. In biomechanical terms, the ability of a sphincteric region to open is related to several factors that include muscle tone, passive viscoelasticity, mechanoreceptor-mediated reflexes, perception and bolus transport [2]. The sphincteric region at the esophagogastric junction (EGJ), commonly known as the lower esophageal sphincter has particularly interested physiologists and gastroenterologists, particularly with regard to its mechanism of action.

Dysfunction of the EGJ allows the reflux of noxious gastric contents such into the esophagus in substantial amounts and for prolonged periods of time [28]. Reflux can be assessed indirectly by measuring the pH in the esophagus. Useful improved techniques for measuring pH in the esophagus [29] and for measuring retrograde flow of stomach contents into the esophagus have recently been developed. Although manometry has long been used to evaluate motility in the esophagus, it has not proven to be consistent in measuring the competence of the EGJ [29]. Until recently no clinical technique has been found really useful to evaluate the EGJ quantitatively.

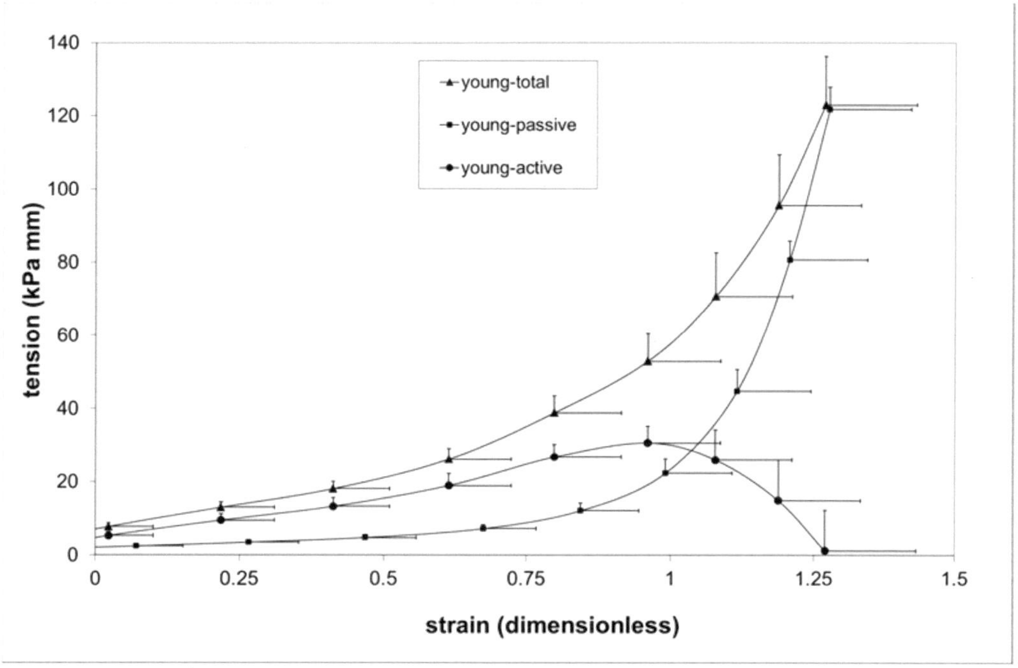

Figure 8: Diagram of active, passive and total tension as function of strain obtained in the gastrointestinal tract of a young human healthy volunteer.

Impedance planimetry has been further developed to form multi-electrode systems for the purpose of measuring a number of cross-sections inside a saline filled bag placed in the human rectum [30]. A sketch of a simple probe with two CSA measurements is shown in Fig. (**5**). McMahon refined the multi-electrode technology in his Ph.D. work, first to three and eight CSAs in the EGJ, and later the technology was commercialized with 16 CSA measurements [31-33]. The development extends the previous work significantly and introduces a novel new method for functionally imaging and evaluating the EGJ and other gastrointestinal sphincters. Basically the probe consists of multiple electrodes inside a bag that spans the whole sphincter including the regions adjacent to it. Distension can be made using various protocols, and the CSAs can be converted to geometric reconstructions of the sphincter as still pictures or as video sequences. Figs. (**9**) and (**10**) show different representations of data obtained in the esophagogastric junction using FLIP.

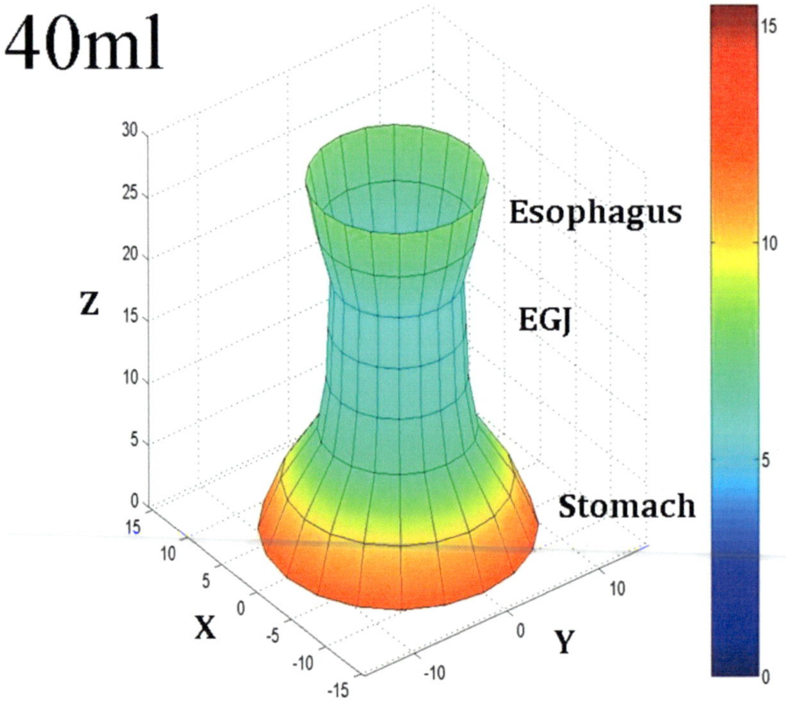

Figure 9: A FLIP generated profile of the EGJ lumen using an 8 CSA channel probe during distension with a volume of 40ml. The widening in the top is the esophageal lumen, the narrow zone is the EGJ and the bottom wide part is inside the fundus of the stomach. X, Y and Z are the three principal axes showing distances (mm) (Courtesy of Professor Barry Mcmanon).

3.4.3. Medical Imaging Technologies

Medical imaging technologies such as MRI, SPECT, and ultrasonography have improved tremendously over the past decades and have proven to be useful in studies of gastric emptying, accommodation and other functions of the gastrointestinal tract. Basically the methods are used to measure volume and how the volume distributes and changes over time. This makes them markedly different from the barostat which is the standard bag technique to measure volume changes at a fixed pressure in the stomach or other organs.

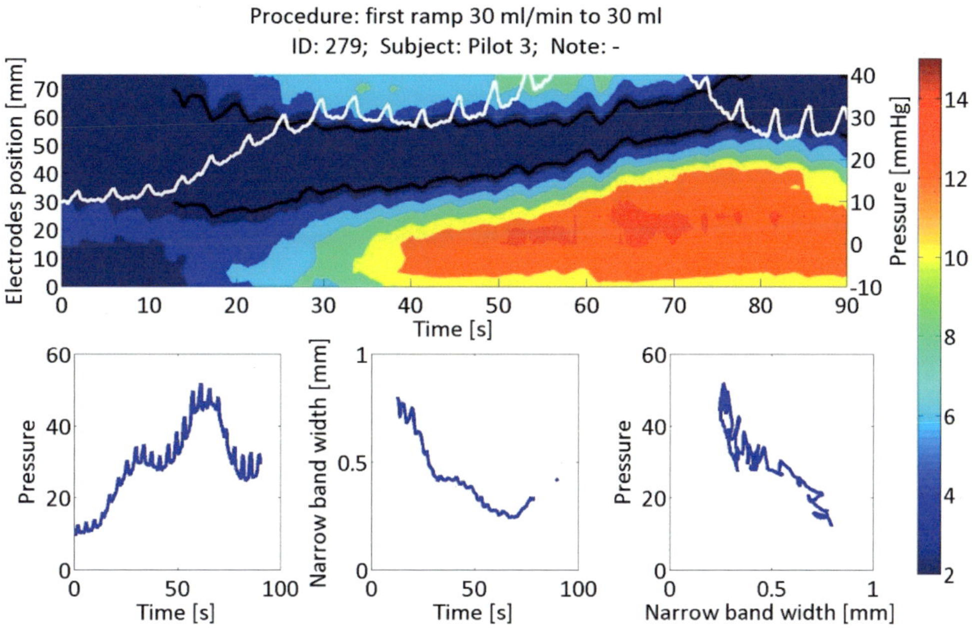

Figure 10: FLIP data from ramp distension in a healthy volunteer expressed a color contour plot based on 16 CSA measurements. The blue zone in the middle of the color plot shows the EGJ (the narrow band). The white tracing is the bag pressure. The color scale to the far right represents diameter magnitude. The pressure and the narrow band width are plotted in the graphs at the bottom.

MRI is an accurate and safe technique for imaging the human stomach [34]. After ingestion of a test meal labelled with gadolinium, images of the gastric region are acquired. The MRI technique permits three-dimensional reconstruction of the stomach, enabling total gastric volume measurements during fasting and postprandially. Single Photon Emission Computed Tomography (SPECT) uses ^{99m}Tc uptake into the gastric mucosa for visualisation and volume estimation of the gastric compartment [35]. Comparison of SPECT data with barostat measurements showed that SPECT is able to detect changes in intragastric volume but unable to detect changes in gastric tone and hence accommodation [36].

The principle of ultrasonography is that short pulses of ultrasound pass through a liquid but are partially reflected by solid interfaces, producing echoes. The depth of the reflecting interface determines the time taken for an echo to return to the ultrasound transducer. A continuous, moving, two-dimensional, image of a slice of tissue is obtained in real-time ultrasonography. The interested reader can find a thorough description of the principles of gastrointestinal ultrasound in Gregersen and Matre [37] and in Ødegaard, Gilja and Gregersen [38].

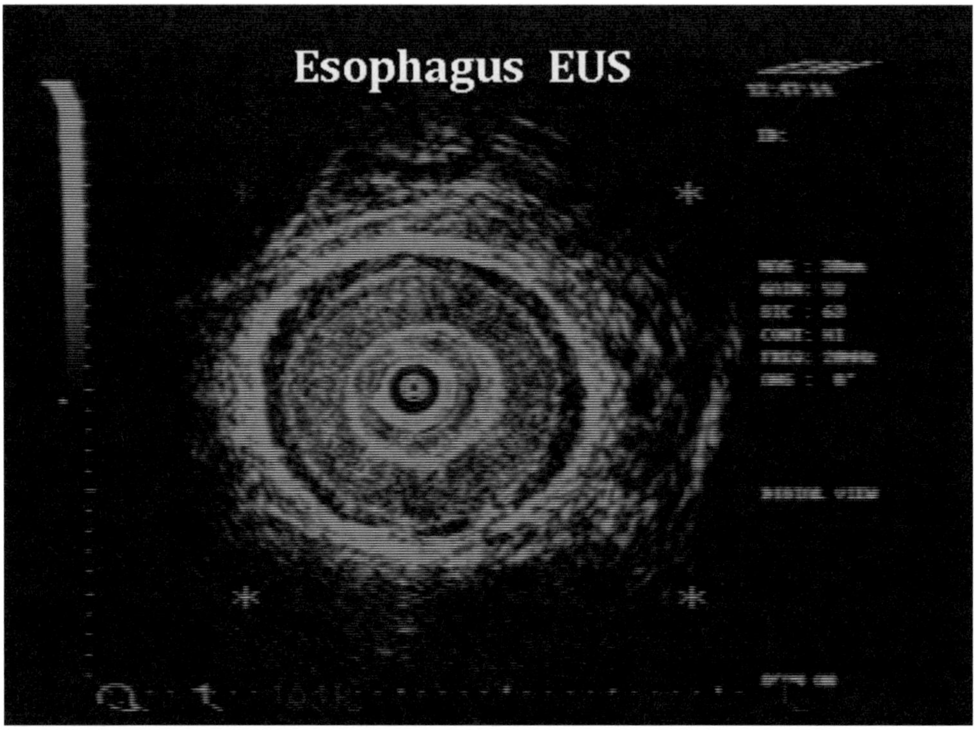

Figure 11: Ultrasonographic image of esophageal wall during a contraction (primary peristalsis). The image is obtained using a 15 MHz endoscopic ultrasound probe in a young volunteer at Haukeland Hospital in Bergen, Norway. Several layers and their interfaces are visible.

Ultrasound in the frequency domain up to 30 MHz can be used *in vivo* using ultrasound endoscopes and provides useful data on the geometry of the cross-section and on the wall thickness (Figs. **11** and **12**). Hence, under certain assumptions and in combination with pressure measurements, it is possible to obtain a value for stress rather than for tension *in vivo*. It is also possible to estimate longitudinal strains from measurement of wall layer areas as devised by Brasseurs group [39]. The ultrasound transducer when scanning from inside the lumen can be placed either on the endoscope on a special probe or on a probe-mounted bag. Furthermore, trans-abdominal scans can be very useful for obtaining geometric data. All techniques are in use by now, though not always with biomechanical purposes in mind. Endoscopic ultrasonography, transabdominal B-mode ultrasonography, and 3D-ultrasonography are useful. However, transabdominal scanning is only possible in some regions of the gastrointestinal tract such as in the antrum. If combined with bag distension, where the pressure is measured and can be controlled, it is possible to compute stress-strain relations *in vivo*.

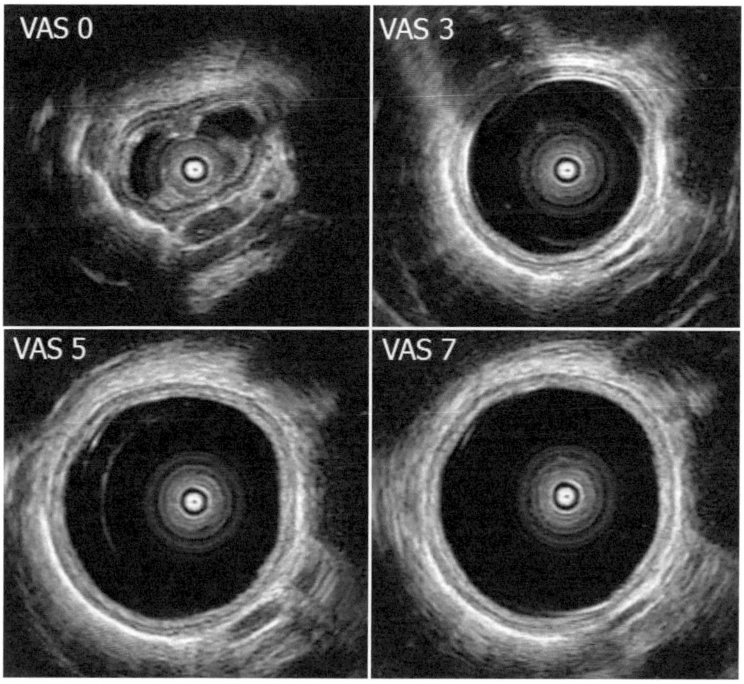

Figure 12: Ultrasonographic images of esophagus in non-distended state (VAS 0) and at distensions to sensory levels of VAS 3, 5 and 7 (using a symptom scale where 0 means no sensation, 5 is the pain threshold and 7 is moderate pain. Wall layers are clearly visible and the esophageal lumen becomes more and more circular at higher degrees of distension. Geometric data obtained from this kind of studies are very useful in biomechanical and mechanosensory studies (Courtesy of Mech-sense).

The different imaging methods exhibit different spatial and temporal image resolution, and these factors strongly influence accuracy in volume calculation. MRI and in particular SPECT imaging have poor spatial and temporal resolution compared to ultrasonography. Ultrasonography provides a good temporal resolution and a spatial resolution on sub-millimeter level. There are few methods that are capable of measuring all parameters of gastric motility simultaneously. However, ultrasonography can be used to study gastric configuration, accommodation, gastric emptying, intragastric distribution, gastric motility, distensibility, transpyloric flow and gastric wall strain [40-46]. The conventional ultrasonography techniques are well known these days, including transabdominal B mode and 3D scanning. In addition to the conventional techniques, elastography and strain rate imaging are emerging as novel techniques. The stiffness of normal and pathological tissue is usually different and may be evaluated by ultrasound which is based on B-mode scanning during compressions (elastography). The underlying principle is that the tissue deformation by a mechanical excitation is a function of its mechanical properties. The intraluminal pressure may be used as the excitation force for gastrointestinal purposes [38]. It is documented as imaged by B-mode ultrasonography that increased pressure on the gastrointestinal wall changes the thickness, layers and echogenicity of the wall [47]. Strain rate imaging is a recent technique to quantitate deformation of biological tissue. Strain rate imaging is based on tissue velocity imaging, which is an ultrasound technique providing quantitative information on velocities within a tissue. With help of color-coded tissue velocity imaging, velocity data from the whole view field are available simultaneously [37]. Hereby extraction of other parameters through spatial and temporal processing of the velocity data can be done. Examples of such parameters are strain rate and strain. These methods have primarily been used in echocardiography. However, other uses have also been reported including measurements of gastric motor function [42].

Endoscopic ultrasonography is of huge interest and deserves further consideration. Intraluminal ultrasonography, also named endo-sonography (ES) or endoscopic ultrasonography (EUS) is the names of ultrasound examinations using transducers inserted into the gastrointestinal tract. The visceral wall and adjacent structures can be viewed in detail. Acoustic coupling can be achieved by filling water into the lumen or into a bag surrounding the ultrasound transducer. Endo-sonography is currently mostly done in the upper gastrointestinal tract and rectum. However, endo-sonographic imaging of the colon and distal ileum as well as intraductal ultrasonography of the biliary and pancreatic ducts are frequently done with miniature probes.

Echo-endoscopes combine integrated ultrasound transducers with endoscopy. The instruments are classified both according to the type of endoscope and the US system. Echo-endoscopes may have radial or curvilinear array US transducers using frequencies between 7.5 and 30 MHz. Doppler sonography provides information about vascular flow and separate vessels from other echo-poor structures. Some echo-endoscopes possess integrated Doppler technology. US miniature probes have a diameter which allows the probe to be inserted through the biopsy channel of a conventional endoscope. Currently, available US miniature probes comprise mechanical sector, electronic phased arrays, or single crystal linear compound systems operating with frequencies between 12 and 30 MHz. The small size and high frequencies of miniature probes reduce the size of the US image and the penetration depth of the US beam into the tissue as compared to echo-endoscopes.

Correct interpretation of ultrasound images of the gastrointestinal wall is important when applying this technique for detailed examination of physiological characteristics. The wall consists of mucosa, submucosa, and circumferential and longitudinal muscle layers separated by the myenteric plexus. The normal gastrointestinal wall is imaged by ultrasonography as a layered structure consisting of 3-9 layers depending on thickness and structure of different layers, ultrasound frequency, and applied pressure on the wall [47, 48]. In some cases, a five-layer structure of the wall can be demonstrated using ES.

Ultrasonography is a useful tool in studies of the geometry and mechanics of the gastrointestinal tract. Nicosia *et al.* (2001) combined manometry and ultrasound and used conservation of mass principles to quantify local axial shortening of the esophagus [39]. A relationship between contractions in the circular and longitudinal muscle layers during swallowing was established. Based on this approach, an association was found between sustained longitudinal layer contraction in the esophageal body and chest pain of unknown origin [49]. Takeda *et al.* (2002) used combined ultrasound and manometry to determine circumferential stress-strain properties in the esophagus [50]. Hoff *et al.* (2006) described a multimodal device for esophagus studies combining bag distension, manometry, high frequency intraluminal ultrasound, laser Doppler flowmetry and symptom registration [51]. Experience indicates that these modalities can be used in combination without significant technical influence on each other.

3.4.4. The Use of Modeling

3.4.4.1. Numerical Methods

The complex geometry of the gastrointestinal tract often requires a number of simplifying assumptions in order to use the theory outlined in chapter 2. If the geometry is complex or valid assumptions cannot be made, we must turn to numerical methods. The most important numerical methods for the approximate solution of partial differential equations problems are the finite difference methods and the finite element methods. One of the advantages of finite element methods is their high flexibility and high efficiency in dealing with irregularly shaped boundaries. It is useful for many gastrointestinal mechanical problems. Examples are

- computation of stresses in esophageal buckles,
- computation of stresses in the vicinity of the mechanosensitive elements in the wall,

- interaction between the fluid motion and the wall motion in peristalsis,
- localized flows in the small intestine.

The numerical methods require the derivation of the desired form of the equations, the choice of a suitable mesh, the development of the finite element form of the equations, and the procedure for solution, and determination of the stability of the resultant algebraic scheme. In finite element analysis, the domain to be analyzed is divided into elements and the displacement field within each element is interpolated in terms of displacements at a few points around the element boundary. These points are called nodes. The interpolation is done so that the displacement field is continuous across element boundaries. The strain at every point can then be expressed in terms of nodal displacements. It is then required that the associated stresses, through the stress-strain relation, satisfy the principle of virtual work for arbitrary variations of the nodal displacements. This generates numerous equations to be solved by computer.

Part of this chapter has been previously published in Neurogastroenterology and motility, volume 12, issue 6, pages 501-508, 2000.

REFERENCES

[1] Cannon WB. The mechanical factors of digestion. Oxford 1911.
[2] Gregersen H. Biomechanics of the Gastrointestinal Tract. Springer Verlag, London 2002.
[3] Hausken T, Odegaard S, Matre K, Berstad A. Antroduodenal motility and movements of luminal contents studied by duplex sonography. Gastroenterology 1992; 102: 1583-90.
[4] Rouillon JM, Azpiroz F, Malagelada JR. Reflex changes in intestinal tone: relationship to perception. Am J Physiol 1991; 261: G280-G286.
[5] Bell AM, Pemberton JH, Hanson RB, Zinsmeister AR. Variations in muscle tone of the human rectum: recordings with an electromechanical_barostat. Am J Physiol 1991; 260: G17-G25.
[6] Gregersen H, Andersen MB. Impedance measuring system for quantification of cross-sectional area in the gastrointestinal tract. Med Biol Eng Comput 1991; 29: 108-110.
[7] Harris JH, Therkelsen EE & Zinner NR. Electrical measurement of ureteral flow. In: Boyarsky S, Tanagho EA, Gottschalk CW & Zimskind PD, Eds. Urodynamics. London, Academic Press 1971; pp. 465-472.
[8] Fisher MA, Hendrix TR, Hunt IN & Murrills AJ. Relation between volume swallowed and velocity of the bolus ejected from the pharynx into the esophagus. Gastroenterology 1978; 74: 1238-1240.
[9] Fass J, Silny J, Braun J, Heindrichs U, Dreuw B, Schumpelick V & Rau G. Ein neues verfahren zur quantitativen bestimmung oesophagealer motilitlltsmuster mittels einer vielfachen impedanzmessung. In: Chirurgiches forum 1989 f. experim. u. kliniche forschung (Ed. Hamelmann *et al*). Springer-Verlag, Berlin 1989.
[10] Colstrup H, Mortensen SO & Kristensen JK. A probe for measurements of related values of cross-sectional area and pressure in the resting female urethra. Urol Res 1983; 11: 139-143.
[11] Colstrup H. Rigidity of the resting female urethra. Part II. Dynamic measurements. J Urol 1984; 132: 82-86.
[12] Lose G, Colstrup H. Mechanical properties of the urethra in healthy and stress incontinent females: dynamic measurements in the resting urethra. J urol 1990; 144: 1258-1262.
[13] Gregersen H, Stødkilde-Jørgensen H, Djurhuus JC, Mortensen SO. The four electrode impedance technique: a method for investigation of compliance in luminal organs. Clin Phys Physiol Meas 1988;9(Suppl. A):61-64.

[14] Gregersen H, Barlow J, Thompson DG. Development of a computer-controlled tensiometer for real-time measurements of tension in tubular organs. Neurogastroenterol Motility 1999; 11: 109-118.

[15] Drewes AM, Schipper KP, Dimcevski G, Petersen P, Andersen OK, Gregersen H, Arendt-Nielsen L. Multimodal induction and assessment of allodynia and hyperalgesia in the human oesophagus. Eur J Pain 2003; 7: 539-549.

[16] Accarino AM, Azpiroz F, Malagelada JR. Symptomatic responses to stimulation of sensory pathways in the jejunum. Am J Physiol 1992; 263: G673-G677.

[17] Fass R, Naliboff B, Higa L, Johnson C, Kodner A, Munakata J, Ngo J, Mayer EA. Differential effect of long-term esophageal acid exposure on mechanosensitivity and chemosensitivity in humans. Gastroenterology 1998; 115: 1363-1373.

[18] Drewes AM, Schipper KP, Dimcevski G, Petersen P, Andersen OK, Gregersen H, Arendt-Nielsen L. Multimodal_assessment of pain in the esophagus: a new experimental model. Am J Physiol 2002; 283: G95-G103.

[19] Reddy H, Staahl C, Arendt-Nielsen L, Gregersen H, Drewes AM, Funch-Jensen P. Sensory and biomechanical properties of the esophagus in non-erosive reflux disease. Scand J Gastroenterol 2007; 42; 432-440.

[20] Drewes AM, Pedersen J, Reddy H, Rasmussen K, Funch-Jensen P, Arendt-Nielsen L, Gregersen H. Central sensitization in patients with non-cardiac chest pain: A clinical experimental pain study. World J Gastroenterol 2006; 41: 640-649.

[21] Krarup AL, Olesen SS, Funch-Jensen P, Gregersen H, Drewes AM. Proximal and distal esophageal sensitivity is decreased in patients with Barrett's esophagus. World J Gastroenterol 2011; 17: 514-21.

[22] Gao C, Arendt-Nielsen L, Liu W, Petersen P, Drewes AM, Gregersen H. Sensory and biomechanical responses to ramp-controlled distension of the human duodenum. Am J Physiol 2003; 284: G461-G471.

[23] Gregersen H, Gilja OH, Hausken T, Heimdal A, Gao C, Matre K, Odegaard S, Berstad A. Mechanical properties in the human gastric antrum using B-mode ultrasonography and antral distension. Am J Physiol 2002; 283: G368-G375.

[24] Guyton AC, Hall JE. Heart muscle. the heart is a pump. In Textbook of Medical Physiology. WB Saunders Company 2002.

[25] Pedersen J, Drewes AM, Gregersen H. New analysis for the study of the muscle function in the human oesophagus. Neurogastroenterol Motil 2005; 17; 767-772

[26] Zhao J, Liao D, Yang J, Gregersen H. Stress and strain analysis of contractions during ramp distension in partially obstructed guinea pig jejunal segments. J Biomech 2011;44: 2077-82.

[27] Liao D, Villadsen GE, Gregersen H. Distension Evoked Motility Analysis in Human Esophagus. Neurogastroenterol Motil. 2013; 25: 407-e297.

[28] Kahrilas PJ. Anatomy and physiology of the gastroesophageal junction. Gastroenterol Clin North Am 1997; 26: 467-86.

[29] Pandolfino JE, Kahrilas PJ. Prolonged pH Monitoring. Bravo Capsule Gastrointest Endosc Clin N Am 2005; 15: 307-318.

[30] Andersen IS, Gregersen H, Buntzen S, Djurhuus JC, Laurberg S. New probe for the measurement of dynamic changes in the rectum. Neurogastroenterol Motil 2004; 16: 99-105.

[31] McMahon BP, Frøkier JB, Drewes AM, Gregersen H. A new measurement of oesophago-gastric junction competence. Neurogastroenterol Motil 2004; 16: 543-546.

[32] McMahon BP, Frøkjær JB, Kunwald P, Donghua L, Funch-Jensen P, Drewes AM, Gregersen H. The Functional Lumen Imaging Probe (FLIP) for Evaluation of the Esophagogastric Junction. Am J Physiol 2007; 292; G377-G384.

[33] Kwiatek M, Kahrilas PJ, Soper N, Bulsiewicz W, McMahon B, Gregersen H, Pandolfino, J. Esophagogastric junction distensibility after fundoplication assessed with a novel functional luminal imaging probe. J Gastrointest Surg 2010; 14: 268-276.

[34] Schwizer W, Steingotter A, Fox M, Zur T, Thumshirn M, Bosiger P, *et al.* Non-invasive measurement of gastric accommodation in humans. Gut 2002; 51: i59-i62.

[35] Kuiken SD, Samsom M, Camilleri M, Mullan BP, Burton DD, Kost LJ, *et al.* Development of a test to measure gastric accommodation in humans. Am J Physiol 1999; 277: G1217-G1221.

[36] van den Elzen BD, Bennink RJ, Wieringa RE, Tytgat GN, Boeckxstaens GE. Fundic accommodation assessed by SPECT scanning: comparison with the gastric barostat. Gut 2003; 52: 1548-54.

[37] Gregersen H, Matre K. The use of Ultrasound in Biomechanics. In: Odegaard S, Gilja OH, Gregersen H. Eds. Basic and New aspects of Gastrointestinal Ultrasonography. Singapore, World Scientific Publishers 2005.

[38] Ødegaard S, Gilja OH, Gregersen H. Basic and New aspects of Gastrointestinal Ultrasonography. Singapore: World Scientific Publishers 2005.

[39] Nicosia MA, Brasseur JG, Liu JB, Miller LS. Local longitudinal muscle shortening of the human esophagus from high-frequency ultrasonography. Am J Physiol 2001; 281: G1022-G1033.

[40] Whittingham TA, Bateman DN. Measurement of stomach volume by real-time ultrasound. Ultrasound Med Biol 1983; 2: 459-63.

[41] Gilja OH, Detmer PR, Jong JM, Leotta DF, Li X-N, Beach KW, *et al.* Intragastric distribution and gastric emptying assessed by 3D-ultrasonography. Gastroenterology 1997; 113: 38-49.

[42] Gilja OH, Heimdal A, Hausken T, Gregersen H, Matre K, Berstad A, Ødegaard S. Strain during gastric contractions can be measured using Doppler ultrasonography. Ultrasound Med Biol 2002; 28: 1457-1465

[43] Hausken T, Berstad A. Wide gastric antrum in patients with non-ulcer dyspepsia. Effect of cisapride. Scand J Gastroenterol 1992; 27: 427-32.

[44] King PM, Adam RD, Pryde A, McDicken WN, Heading RC. Relationships of human antroduodenal motility and transpyloric fluid movement. non-invasive observations with real-time ultrasound. Gut 1984; 25: 1384-91.

[45] Liao D, Gregersen H, Hausken T, Gilja OH, Mundt M, Kassab G. Analysis of surface geometry of the human stomach using real-time 3-D ultrasonography *in vivo*. Neurogastroenterol Motil 2004; 16: 315-24.

[46] Matre K, Ahmed A, Gregersen H, Heimdal A, Hausken T, Odegaard S, *et al. In vitro* evaluation of ultrasound Doppler strain rate imaging. Modification for measurement in slow moving tissue phantom. Ultrasound Med Biol 2003; 29: 1725-34.

[47] Ødegaard S, Kimmey MB, Martin RW, Yee HC, Cheung AHS, Silverstein FE. The effects of applied pressure on the thickness, layers, and echogenicity of gastrointestinal wall ultrasound images. Gastrointest Endosc 1992; 38: 351-6.

[48] Kimmey MB, Martin RW, Haggitt RC, Wang KY, Franklin DW, Silverstein FE. Histological correlates of gastrointestinal endoscopic ultrasound images. Gastroenterology 1989; 96: 433-441.

[49] Balaban DH, Yamamoto Y, Liu J, Pehlivanov N, Wisniewski R, DeSilvey D, Mittal RK. Sustained esophageal contraction, a marker of esophageal chest pain identified by intraluminal ultrasonography. Gastroenterology 1999; 116: 29-37.

[50] Takeda T, Kassab G, Liu J, Puckett JL, Mittal RR, Mittal RK. A novel ultrasound technique to study the biomechanics of the human esophagus *in vivo*. Am J Physiol 2002; 282: G785-G793.

[51] Hoff DA, Gregersen H, Odegaard S, Nesje LB, Oevreboe K, Hausken T, Gilja OH, Matre K, Hatlebakk JG. A multimodal laser Doppler and endosonographic distention device for studying mechanosensation and mucosal blood flow in the oesophageus. Neurogastroenterol Motil 2006; 18: 243-248

CHAPTER 4

The Mechanical System: Muscle and Connective Tissue

Abstract: A number of factors affect neuromuscular function in the gastrointestinal tract and so act upon the transport of material. The intrinsic properties of the muscle account for the mechanics. These properties of the muscle itself establish the relationships between length, tension and velocity. This chapter deals primarily with the tissue properties, both active and passive, of the gastrointestinal wall. It seems obvious that the passive properties are related to non-contractile elements where the active properties are due to the contraction of the smooth muscle cells. Hill's three-element model explains the active and passive elements in the wall and their interaction.

Keywords: Connective tissue, gastrointestinal muscle, Hill′s model, large intestine, oesophagus, passive properties, small intestine, sphincters, stomach, zero-stress state.

4.1. INTRODUCTION

The motor function of the gastrointestinal tract seems to be at first glance perplexing and unpredictable in comparison to other areas of systemic physiology. There seems to be no scheme of the whole system that is grounded in the rational interpretation of experimental observation. Such a perspective could provide a theory to be used both to interpret the variety of normal or usual behaviors and to predict the responses to exceptional conditions. However, our relative ignorance about gastrointestinal motor physiology continues to allow only superficial interpretations and predictions in health and disease.

The empiricism surrounding so much of gastrointestinal motility derives from the complexity of the biological and the physical processes, both in the muscle and in the mechanics. A number of factors affect neuromuscular function in the gastrointestinal tract and so act upon the transport of material. The nervous factors determine especially the topology, frequency, and time sequence of contraction. The intrinsic properties of the muscle account for the mechanics. These properties of the muscle itself establish the relationships between length, tension and velocity.

This chapter deals primarily with the tissue properties, both active and passive, of the gastrointestinal wall. It seems obvious that the passive properties are related to non-contractile elements where the active properties are due to the contraction of the smooth muscle cells. Hill's three-element model, developed many years ago, explains the active and passive elements in the wall and their interaction [1].

Hans Gregersen and James Christensen

4.2. HILL'S THREE-ELEMENT MODEL

The three-dimensional distribution of stress and strain in the gastrointestinal tract and the effect of strain and stress on the biology of the longitudinal and circumferential muscle layers, the submucosa, and the mucosa have not been studied in detail. For this reason, the overall scheme must be briefly covered here. Since the active muscle contraction is the most important feature of the peristaltic movement of the gastrointestinal tract, the way in which the muscle is considered in theory must be described first.

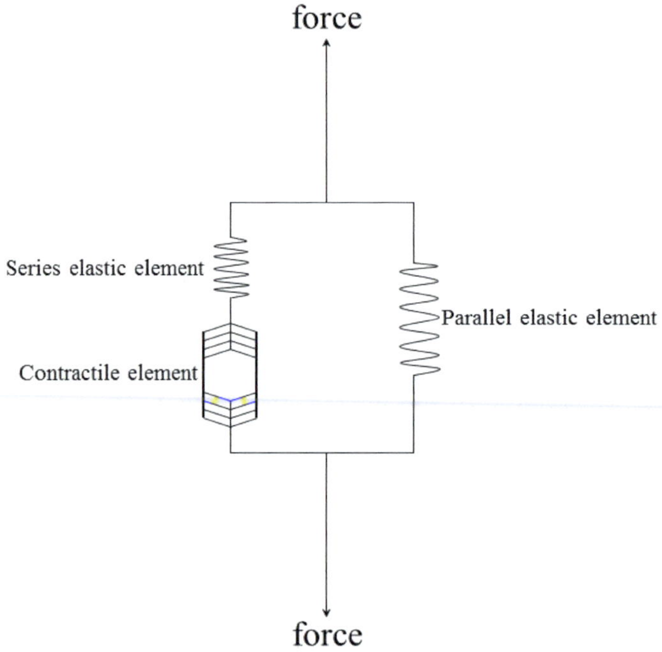

Figure 1: Illustration of Hill's model with the three elements. The parallel element represents the connective tissues and the quiescent muscle cells. The contractile element represents the active contraction, shortening and tension generation machinery. The series element represents the elasticity of actin and myosin fibers and cross-bridges.

The "three element model" of the Nobel Laureate, A.V. Hill, from 1939, considers muscle tissue as composed of a "contractile element" connected with a "series elastic element" for describing the active contraction of the muscle, and a "parallel element" for describing the connective tissue (such as collagen, elastin and other matrix molecules) (Fig. **1**). This model has been applied in numerous studies to heart, lung, blood vessels, and kidney mechanics. Many modifications have been made, yet no competing model had a better success in explaining the range of behaviors.

Applying the Hill model to the gastrointestinal tract, we consider as "parallel elements" the mucosa, the submucosa and the quiescent muscles whereas the contractile and series elastic elements belong to the active muscle. The contractile element is identical to the sliding actin-myosin molecules. At rest, there is no tension in this element but active tension is generated when the number of cross-bridges increases. From isometric experiments (see chapter 2 and 3 and later in this chapter), it is known that an optimum sarcomere length exists where the active tension has its maximum. The number of cross-bridges explains this feature. When the muscle is elongated too much, the actin and myosin molecules are pulled too far apart and the number of possible cross-bridges decreases. If the muscle is shortened too much, the actin filaments interfere with each other. If we assume that the contractile element does not contribute tension in the resting state, then the stress-strain-history of the resting muscle determines the constitutive equation of the parallel element. Hence, the difference between the mechanical properties of the whole muscle and those of the parallel element characterizes the combination of the contractile and series elastic elements.

Because of the coupling in series between these two elements, the division of the strain between these elements is not unique. On basis of the further assumptions that must be made, Fung provided the equations for a number of experimental conditions and also pointed the limitations of Hill's model [2]. It is pointed out above that the contraction of a muscle depends on its precontractile length. Since the body is a very efficient device for saving energy, one may expect the gastrointestinal tract to use mechanisms to bring the muscle into the optimal position or condition for contraction. In the gastrointestinal tract, the smooth muscle cells are oriented both circumferentially and longitudinally, and small changes in their contractile state may considerably change the geometry of the lumen and the wall stiffness. In that respect, Christensen and Macagno described long ago that longitudinal contractions in the small intestine causes specific flow patterns to mix the fluids, and that they increase the diameter of the intestine, which may affect its distensibility [3]. Pal and Brasseur showed that the longitudinal contraction in the esophagus that often precedes a circular contraction serve to put the circular muscle layer in a position to contract with greater force [4]. The rationale is that the longitudinal contraction thickens the wall and, according to Laplace's law, this creates a higher pressure during the circular muscle contraction than would occur from a circular contraction without a preceding contraction in the longitudinal muscle layer.

The effect of the tissue properties during loading and the zero-stress state on physiologic functions may not be clear until the full Hill's model is analyzed. But it is clear that the zero-stress state (see later in this chapter) and the mechanical properties of collagen and other matrix components are fundamental features of the parallel element.

The parallel element is important for the function of the contractile element. For example, the muscle cell length depends on the strain of the parallel element. Hence, whether or not the muscle can achieve the optimum length of the length-tension relationship for its contraction depends on strain related to the zero-stress state of the parallel element [2]. Hill's three-element model helps explain the interaction between the parallel and contractile elements. Further work is needed to determine how the residual stress and strains affect the responses to physical and chemical stimulation in pathophysiological states.

Since the gastrointestinal tract is essentially a muscular tube, any alteration of the activity of the smooth muscle cells by agents acting on the muscles directly or on their innervation changes the mechanical state of this organ. Hence, the effects of such agents on the gastrointestinal tract need investigation in order to model accurately the normal bolus transport in health and disease.

4.3. PASSIVE MECHANICAL PROPERTIES

Using Hill's model, we can now explain what determines the shape of the distensibility curves. Smooth muscle contributes to the distensibility both passively (through the abundance and nature of the extracellular collagen in the muscle) and actively (through contraction). Though it is not difficult to record contractile activity *in vitro* and *in vivo*, it is easier to analyze and interpret the passive performance of the tissue, such as that present during the administration of smooth muscle relaxants. As pointed out in the previous section about Hill's model, the understanding of the passive behavior of gut smooth muscle is also a prerequisite for understanding its active behavior. Therefore, the passive state that can be studied *in vitro* (and to some extent *in vivo*) will be considered first.

It is well known that the passive elastic behavior of biological tissues is non-linear (exponential-like). This mechanical feature protects the tissue against supra-physiological distension and damage at high luminal pressure loads and wall stresses while allowing the organ to distend easily at lower loads, and thus this characteristic facilitates flow in the physiological pressure range. It has been shown in arteries that collagen bears circumferential loads at high stress levels.

Due to the richness of collagen in gastrointestinal tissue, collagen seems most likely to be the major determinant of its passive properties.

Only few data exist on the relation between elastic properties and morphology in the gastrointestinal tract. Fackler *et al.* [5] and Orberg *et al.* [6] showed the bi-axial orientation of collagen fibers in the submucosa (where it forms a framework constituting both clockwise and counterclockwise helices with a 30-degree angle between them). They also demonstrated how the fibers uncrimp (unfold) at low levels of stress rather than being stretched. Other studies have demonstrated a correlation between the total collagen content and the biomechanical properties in experimental models involving partial obstruction of the gut. It is also known that collagen deficiency changes the passive mechanics (studied primarily at the zero-stress state).

The stress-strain relation depends mainly on the passive elastic properties of tissue (the elastic properties should be properly called "pseudoelastic" because loading and unloading curves follow different paths). According to the Hill model, the curve reflect the properties of the parallel elastic component, which is believed to be anatomically located in the abundant collagen mass in the connective tissue, since the contractile element of smooth muscle by itself does not contribute significantly to the passive tension.

Although it is more difficult to study the passive properties *in vivo* due to contractility and the difficulty in quantitation of the transmural pressure, phasic contractions can, to a variable degree, be greatly reduced in experiments *in vivo* by the administration of drugs such as butylscopolamine. A lowering degree of contractile activity facilitates the differentiation of passive and active properties. If phasic contractions are present, the passive tension (assuming Laplace's law is valid) can be evaluated in the intervals between contractions, where inertial forces can be neglected. However, active properties such as specific tone may still be present. Specific tone may cause a shift at the lower end of the tension-strain curves and consequently may be difficult to differentiate from the passive properties. Animal studies are required to assess the possible contribution of tone, for validation of the baseline pressure determination, and for evaluating the contribution of tethering to the transmural pressure in the distended organ wall.

As explained above, the passive properties in gastrointestinal tissue are primarily due to the properties of the abundant collagen in the wall. There are, however, important differences between the various gastrointestinal organs in the amount of collagen. The esophagus contains a very thick submucosa, whereas the submucosa in the small intestine is thin but nevertheless very strong.

Before reviewing the data in the literature on the stress-strain properties in the gastrointestinal tract (primarily obtained in animal experimental models), we must introduce the concept of the zero-stress state.

4.4. THE ZERO-STRESS STATE OF THE GASTROINTESTINAL TRACT

It is necessary to know the stress-strain relationships of the tissues to understand the tissue forces in the gastrointestinal tract. The stress-strain relationships must be computed in reference to the zero-stress state (the condition where neither external nor internal forces deform the tissue). The basic equations for computing stress and strain are given in Chapter 2.

The zero-stress state of the tissue constitutes the standard state for describing tissue morphology because the tissue is not deformed by internal and external forces. The residual stress and strain cannot be assessed if the zero-stress state is not known. Hence the determination of the zero-stress state of gastrointestinal tissue is the first step in the discovery of its mechanical properties.

The zero-stress state of an organ is the state in which the organ is free of stress, in other words that all external and internal forces are non-existing. Until 1983, it was believed that biological organs were stress-free when all external loads were removed (now defined as the no-load state). In 1983, Fung and Vaishnav and Vossoughi reported independently that the no-load state of a blood vessel is not stress-free (For detailed descriptions and reviews see [2, 7-10]). This was demonstrated by an experiment in which it was seen that rings of arteries after making a radial cut opened up into sectors. The differences in stress and in strain between the no-load (Fig. **2**, top) and zero-stress state (Fig. **2**, bottom) were called the residual stress and the residual strain, respectively. It was discovered that the opening angle of the sector was a way to quantitate the residual stress (Fig. **2**). Fig. (**2**) shows the no-load and zero-stress states schematically, whereas Fig. (**3**) shows photographs of small intestinal segments in the no-load and zero-stress states, demonstrating a somewhat more complex geometry that the schematics shown in Fig. (**2**). Since 1983 numerous studies have been done on the zero-stress state in different organ systems.

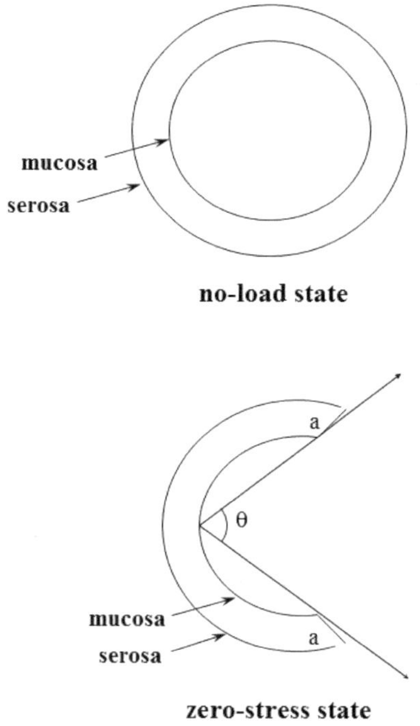

Figure 2: Schematic drawing of cross-section of a gastrointestinal specimen in no-load state and zero-stress state. The zero-stress state is characterized by an opening angle θ which is the angle subtended by two radii drawn to the inner tips of two ends of the sector from the mid-point of the inner wall in the zero-stress state. a is the line of cutting.

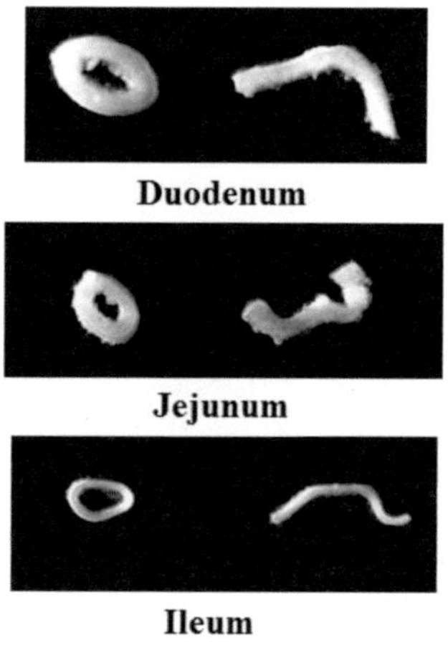

Figure 3: Photographs showing small intestinal specimens in the no-load state (closed ring) and in the zero-stress state (zero-bending moment state). The tissue was obtained from rats. Radial cuts in the tissue rings caused it to spring open, but not into a sectors which could be characterized by opening angles (pictures kindly provided by Professor Jingbo Zhao).

The first data on residual strains and stresses in the gastrointestinal tract was published in 1996 by Gregersen and Kassab [9]. We realize now that the gastrointestinal zero-stress configuration is very different from that of the no-load condition. Furthermore, the zero-stress state is sensitive to growth and remodeling. These studies have opened up a whole new field in relation to gastrointestinal physiology and pathophysiology. Data have been quickly emerging during the last decade. Data have been published on the zero-stress state of the esophagus, the small intestine, the large intestine and the biliary tract in normal animals and in animals exposed to different experimental conditions and diseases. The stomach and the sphincteric regions still lack thorough studies in this way.

4.4.1. How to Access the Zero-Stress State

Zero-stress state experiments must be done under standardized conditions *in vitro*. The excised gastrointestinal segments are cleaned of the luminal contents and the adjacent tissue is dissected away. The segment is transferred to an organ bath containing Krebs solution. Often, the solution that is used is calcium-free and contains a relaxant drug such as EGTA to chelate intracellular calcium stores under otherwise physiological experimental conditions. This achieves the greatest possible relaxation of the muscle, eliminating as far as possible the ability of the muscle to contract. The elimination of muscle activity is important because muscle contraction may affect the passive zero-stress state.

The method is simple. For a tubular organ, two cuts made transverse to the longitudinal axis of the tube will produce a ring. This ring will open into a sector when it is cut radially. Often 30 minutes or more are needed before a stable opening angle is reached.

4.4.2. How to Quantitate the Residual Stresses and Strain

For establishing the zero-stress state, it is necessary to make a sufficient number of cuts for elimination of the internal stresses and strains. The zero-stress state for a tubular organ is an open sector that is defined by an opening angle. Fig. (**2**) (bottom) shows schematically a circumferential tissue sector in the stress-free state. The angle is named the opening angle **θ**, defined as the subtended angle between the two radii from the midpoint of the arc of the inner wall of the intestinal ring to the inner tips of the sector.

Other measures than the opening angle exist to reflect the circumferential residual stress in the tissue. Measures such as the tangent rotation angle and the angle between the tip tangents may be more appropriate measures when the residual stresses are very large and when the cross-section is not circular such as those observed in Fig. (**3**). Still other measures were developed to describe the residual stresses in other directions than the circumferential direction. The interested reader can read more about these measures elsewhere [9-14].

So far, only angle measurements have been considered here. Strain measurements, however, are fundamental in mechanical studies. As discussed in Chapter 2, strain describes the mechanical deformation of a material. In a distensible biological tube like the gastrointestinal tract, the strain of principal interest is the circumferential strain. The loaded *in vivo* strain of the mucosa and serosa must be computed in reference to the mucosal and serosal circumferential lengths at zero-stress. In the esophagus (because of its thick submucosa), it may also be possible to measure the length of the interface between the mucosa-submucosa and the muscle layers. For a continuum subjected to finite deformation, strain can be defined in several different ways in relation to the deformation gradient. The equations given in chapter 2 are to be used where the reference length is simply the length measured at the zero-stress state. For example, the equation for the Cauchy strain relative to the zero-stress state at the mucosal surface is defined as

$$\varepsilon_{\text{mucosa}} = \frac{C_{l-mu\cos a} - C_{z-mu\cos a}}{C_{z-mu\cos a}} \qquad (4.1)$$

where C is the length of distance between any two neighboring material particles. Subscripts *l* and *Z* refer to the loaded and zero-stress states, respectively. If the loaded state is replaced by the no-load state, the strains are called residual strains. Thus, from the circumferential lengths in the no-load state, the loaded state and the zero-stress state, we can compute the circumferential residual or loaded strain, respectively, at the mucosal and serosal surfaces (or at any interface where we can measure the length of the interface) either in the sense of Cauchy or Green. Negative strain implies that the tissue is in compression whereas positive strain implies extension.

It is worthwhile to note that esophagus is the only known organ in the body where the muscle layers can be separated from the mucosa-submucosa layer without apparent damage to the layers. This gives an excellent opportunity to study geometric configuration and zero-stress states of individual layers. Fig. (**4**) shows a sketch of tissues in loaded state, no-load state, intact wall zero-stress state and individual layer zero-stress state and Fig. (**5**) shows an esophageal specimen in no-load, intact wall zero-stress state and separated layer zero-stress state.

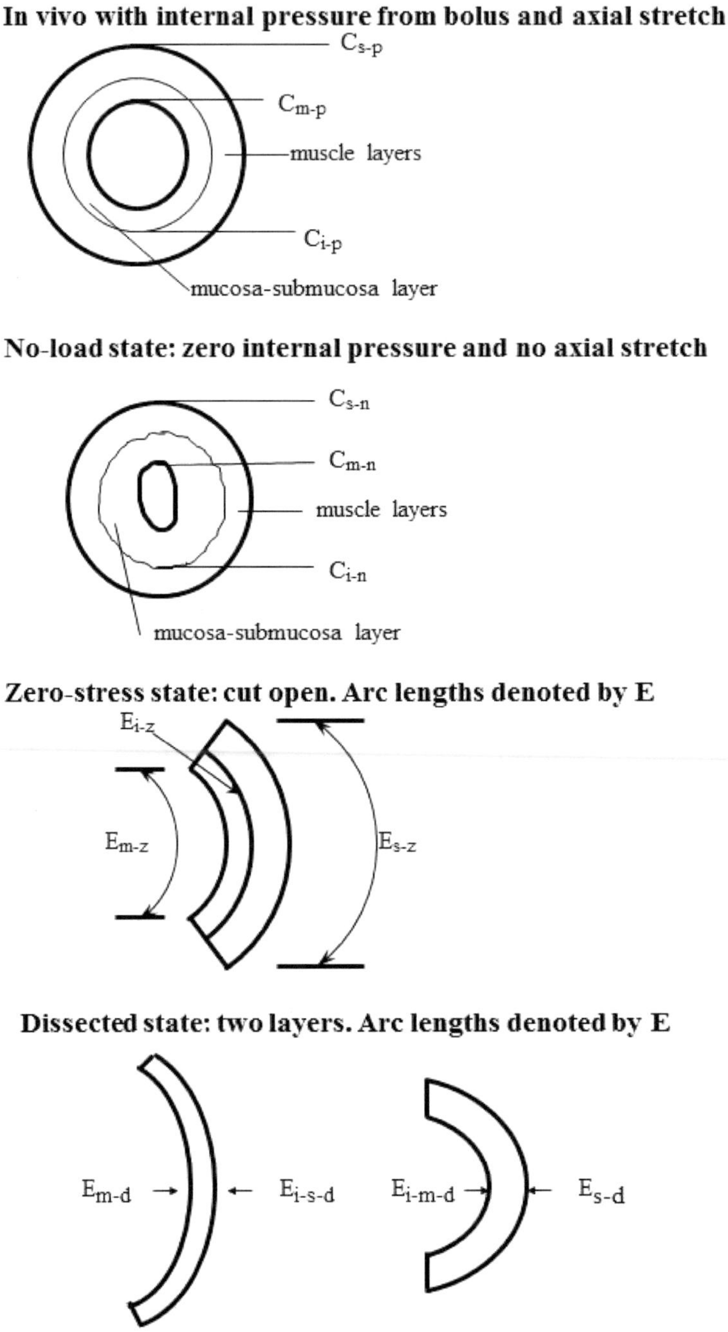

Figure 4: Sketch of an esophageal specimen at various loaded, unloaded and zero-stress states. C is circumferential length and E is arc length. N and z are no-load and zero-stress state. s, I and m indicate serosa, interface and mucosa, respectively (Modified from [13]).

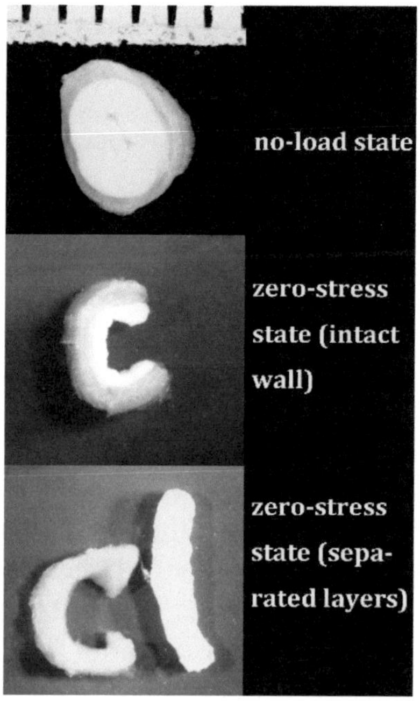

Figure 5: An esophageal specimen at no-load and two well-defined zero-stress states.

4.4.3. Implications of Residual Strain

The existence of the zero-stress state has several important implications, some of which are still hypothetical. From the above discussion is it evident that the use of any state other than the zero-stress state will lead to errors in stress and strain computations. An analysis of strain must refer to the zero-stress state in order for specimens obtained from different locations in the gastrointestinal tract or from different species to be compared. It is also mandatory in any investigation of the remodeling induced by diseases, growth or degeneration. All studies done thus far in the gastrointestinal tract show that the rings open into sectors when cut radially. In fact, tissues from the guinea-pig small intestine have presented the largest residual stresses observed in any tissue thus far.

The following statements summarize some conclusions about the zero-stress state and residual strain. The following paragraphs indicate some of their implications in respect to the motor function of the gastrointestinal tract:

- The zero-stress state is a standard state for describing gastrointestinal tissue morphology since it is not influenced by external or internal forces that deform the tissue.

- Residual strains strengthen the tissue (just as residual strains do in prestressed engineering materials).

- Residual strain influences the resistance to bolus flow because peristaltic bolus transport tends to bulge out the wall (at least in the esophagus).

- The residual tension in the muscle may serve to provide an optimum length for muscle contraction.

- The mucosa is being compressed in the no-load state (and in the low pressure physiological range). Consequently, the stress concentrations at the inner wall of the gastrointestinal tract at no-load and homeostatic states are reduced by the residual stress. Therefore, the compressed mucosa is at least in theory better protected against injury from the flow of luminal contents than uncompressed mucosa is. These protective mechanisms could be important when pathophysiologically high pressures are reached, for example, as recorded in mechanical obstruction.

The mucosal compression produced by the residual forces in the esophagus buckles the mucosa to create the longitudinal folds familiar to the radiologist and gastroenterologist. The gastrointestinal tract uses buckling to advance its normal function. When the lumen is empty, a small tension in the circumferential muscle is sufficient to cause large buckling of the mucosa and submucosa. The esophageal mucosa buckles into a multi-lobed cross-sectional outline. The number of lobes is a characteristic number theoretically computable according to the first principles of mechanics, provided that the constitutive equation (*i.e.*, the stress-strain relationship of the material) is known. For the esophagus, the conditions of buckling are: 1) the tissues are incompressible so that the volume of the tissue remains constant in the process of buckling, and 2) the compressive stresses and strains are small. Hence, the total length of the inner wall of the lumen remains almost constant. These conditions can easily be verified from analysis of photographs of specimens. The equations describing the balance of forces and mass conservation and the minimization of strain energy yield the details of the buckling pattern.

What is the function of the esophageal mucosal buckling? It acts to oppose gastroesophageal reflux. Reflux disease is associated with mucosal inflammation. It is well known that the tone in the lower esophageal sphincter and secondary peristalsis in the esophageal body serve to prevent reflux. However, residual stress causing the mucosal buckling serves as another mechanism to close the esophageal lumen and so oppose the reflux of the gastric contents. The required minimal tension, or tone, in the circumferential muscle to achieve this function can be computed.

In the small intestine, another function of mucosal compression may be important. It is well known that the epithelium, the innermost layer of the mucosa in the small intestine, has the shortest half-life of any system of cells in the body. The very rapid turnover of the mucosal surface may contribute to mucosal compression and hence partly account for the presence of large residual strains.

Conversely, mucosal growth may be affected by the large compressive stresses. Intestinal studies and other organs studies have demonstrated the importance of mechanical stresses for regulating gene expression and growth. Well-known examples from other organs are the cardiac hypertrophy caused by hypertension and the muscle atrophy that occurs in space flight.

Theoretically, the absorption of luminal contents and the secretion of fluids and enzymes may also be dependent on the compression. A gradient in the height of the mucosal villi exists along the small intestine, with the highest villi found in the proximal duodenum, has been described. In various parts of the small intestine, a correlation may exist between the residual strain gradient, the gradient in the height of villi, and the absorption and secretion patterns. These and other testable hypotheses await validation.

Other important issues relate to the function of the mechanoreceptors of the sensory afferent nerves (the intraganglionic laminar endings or other still unknown structures in the gastrointestinal wall). These mechanoreceptors initiate the sensory signals that bring about changes in motor function in the process of self-regulation, one of the critical characteristics of the gastrointestinal motor apparatus. Different receptor classes such as low- and high-threshold mechanoreceptors seem to exist. From physiological studies, not morphological studies, receptors are thought to be located in the submucosa, in the myenteric plexus and in the muscle layers. The stress-free state studies have shown the existence of a strain gradient from the mucosa to the serosa of the wall under physiological conditions. The implication may be that the receptor populations from different locations in the wall will have different zero-settings and therefore will respond differently to the same luminal or external stimuli because of the variation in the magnitudes of distension-induced tensile stresses and strains and in the magnitudes of compressive stresses and strains during contraction. Indeed a difference in the responses of mucosal and muscle mechanoreceptors to stimuli has been observed in some studies. Of course, mechanoreceptor kinetics must be studied *in vivo* under conditions as nearly "normal" as possible. Any change in the geometry of the environment of the mechanoreceptor must be assumed to alter its behavior. The examination of mechanoreceptor kinematics in tissues in any other geometry will likely give erroneous results. Data from all studies of mechanoreceptor kinematics, however, can only be described properly with reference to the zero-stress state.

The zero-stress state is sensitive to remodeling by disease, growth or degeneration. A change in the opening angle of the zero-stress state is a result of non-uniform tissue remodeling of the organ wall. Fung hypothesized that the opening angle increases when the outer layers atrophy more than the inner layers or when the inner layers have a higher growth rate than the outer layers [2, 7]. This has been found largely to be true for the gastrointestinal tract. Rodriguez *et al.* showed by theoretical analysis that volumetric tissue growth alters residual stress [15]. They predicted that *concentric hypertrophy*, characterized by increased wall thickness-to-radius ratio, increases the opening angle and residual stress, and conversely that *eccentric hypertrophy* decreases the opening angle. However, the opening angle of the zero-stress state might not change if homogeneous growth occurs in the tissue. The gastrointestinal wall may be able to remodel itself in such a way as to maintain optimum circumferential stress, although the zero-stress state is a condition that is never experienced *in vivo*. Residual stress or strain also affects the histological changes during remodeling in addition to the mechanical factors, such as intestinal flow (shear) and pressure (circumferential tension),. Residual stress may affect the remodeling by varying the stress distribution in the organ. The data on the residual strains in the gastrointestinal tract and the non-uniform remodeling may be used to improve the results of surgery. For example, procedures might be designed to prestress the tissue to make it more resistant to injury. An additional application may lie in a search for drugs to influence tissue growth and remodeling.

4.5. RESIDUAL STRAIN AND PASSIVE STRESS (TENSION)-STRAIN DATA IN NORMAL TISSUE

Numerous data on residual stress and strain exist from rats, guinea-pigs, rabbits, pigs and humans. Studies in normal animals have been done primarily with the purpose of studying the physiological remodeling during maturation. Studies in humans have been confined mainly to tension-strain experiments using impedance planimetry. However, papers are available on antrum stress-strain distributions as obtained by balloon distension in the antrum and esophagus combined with B-mode ultrasonography.

Summarizing a large number of studies in animals and humans, the mechanical behavior in the gastrointestinal tract is characterized by:

- Nonlinearity of the stress-strain relation. It has, in general, been found that exponential constitutive equations fit the experimental stress-strain relations well (in accord with uniaxial and biaxial constitutive laws).

- Large deformation.

- Large residual stresses and strains in both circumferential and longitudinal directions. The opening angle in the esophagus in most species examined (in all of whom the muscle is striated) is between 60 and 100 degrees, whereas the small intestine has much higher opening angles; the guinea-pig duodenum, in fact, becomes completely inverted, meaning that the opening angle is much larger than 360 degrees.

- Axial variation in the zero-stress state and the stress-strain properties throughout the gastrointestinal tract. The duodenum is stiffer than the more caudal parts of the small intestine. The differences in stiffness likely reflect the specialized functions of the rostral and caudal parts of the small intestine. For example, the duodenum has been proposed to act as a capacitative resistor in gastric emptying, whereas the distal ileum acts rather as a reservoir. Transit slows along the small intestine, and this could be explained partly by the difference in the viscosity of the chyme, but the passive elastic properties may also contribute. A passing bolus might be slowed to a lesser degree in the duodenum where the wall stiffness is high than in the ileum where the compliant ileal wall can bulge a little, allowing and decreased flow.

- Anisotropic mechanical behavior with respect to the circumferential and longitudinal stress–strain relations and to the circumferential and longitudinal zero-stress state. For example, the esophagus is stiffer in the longitudinal direction than in the circumferential direction, at least *in vivo*.

- Differences between the layers (at least in the esophagus, the only organ where this can easily be shown) with the submucosa being the stiffest layer.

4.5.1. Physiological Remodeling in the Esophagus and Intestine during Normal Growth and Maturation

Only a few studies have further examined the zero-stress state and the stress-strain relation during physiological remodeling [16, 17]. Although the origin of residual stress in soft tissues remains uncertain, experimental and theoretical evidence indicates that hypertrophy and geometric remodeling can alter it. Rats aged from 1-32 weeks old have been studied. The opening angle in esophagus was approximately 140 degrees at one and two weeks of age. It gradually decreased to approximately 80 degrees after 16 weeks. Accompanying the geometric shape changes, there was a corresponding significant decrease in opening angle, suggesting that residual strain and stress also decrease with growth. Consistent with the theoretical prediction by Rodriguez *et al.* [15] and many experimental vascular studies, the opening angle correlated with the wall thickness-to-radius ratio. A simple kinematic analysis of uniform transmural growth predicts that the opening angle is proportional to ln (h/r) because the opening angle is determined by the relative change in the thickness-to-radius ratio. At a given circumferential stress, the corresponding strain values became larger up to four weeks of age, whereas after that no further change was observed. That is, the esophagus becomes more compliant during the first four weeks of life. At a given longitudinal stress, the corresponding strain values became larger up to 16 weeks of age after which time no further change was observed. That is, the esophagus becomes more compliant longitudinally during the first 16 weeks after birth. The esophagus was less stiff in the circumferential direction compared to the longitudinal direction.

The remodeling in the small intestine resembled that in the esophagus in the fact that the geometry, the zero-stress state and the stress-strain relation all changed. In particular the small intestine became softer during maturation (Fig. **6**). For the gastrointestinal tract, we must speculate that load increases during physiologic growth will be balanced by appropriate geometric changes to be regulated by a combination of factors. Based on the law of Laplace, the results mentioned above suggest that mean circumferential wall stress increases with age in the rat, since the wall thickness-to-radius ratio decreases substantially, and so stress may play a central role as a regulatory factor. Although the present data do not confirm this hypothesis directly, a stress-dependent growth law can likely be derived that would help to uncover the actual stimulus to hypertrophic tissue growth.

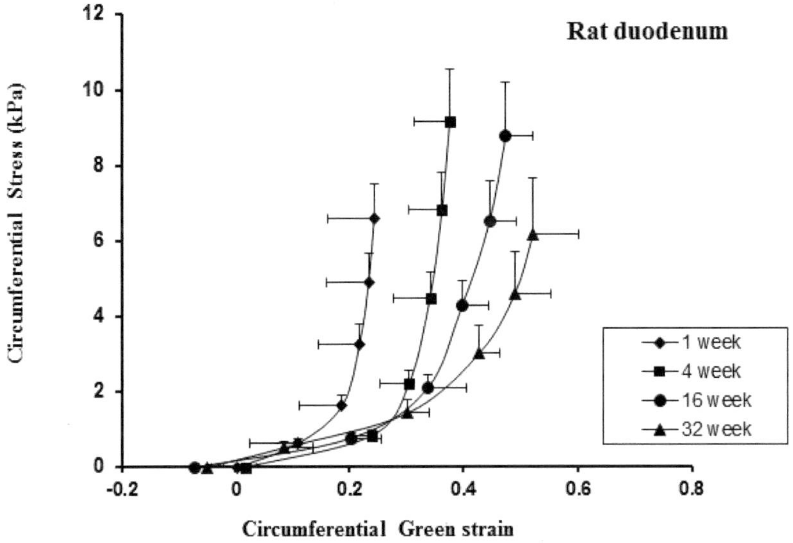

Figure 6: Stress-strain relations of the rat duodenum during maturation process in rats aged 1 week to 32 weeks. The intestine clearly became softer during the period.

4.5.2. Small Intestinal Remodeling during Fasting and Refeeding

This section deals with the remodeling that takes place during fasting and refeeding. Fasting is a common phenomenon in nature. It is part of the normal biological cycle in some animal species and appears during long periods of nutritional deprivation from food shortages caused by natural disasters. Clinically it can result from anorexia, self-imposed food restriction and any serious condition in which feeding is suspended, as in patients nourished mainly or entirely by parenteral means. During fasting, the organism is subjected to a negative nitrogen balance, metabolic changes, and weight loss. It seems obvious that the gastrointestinal tract must also undergo structural and functional adaptation in fasting.

Dou *et al.* studied the changes in the stress-free state and the stress-strain relation of the rat intestine that take place during fasting and refeeding [18, 19]. Rats were fasted for up to 1 week. Other groups of rats were fasted for 1 week and were allowed to survive up to 1 week after refeeding was initiated. The fasted animals lost weight in a linear fashion during the fasting period. The re-fed animals regained the lost weight after 7 days of re-feeding. The duodenum seems to experience the greatest loss during fasting, for the duodenal weight-to-length ratio gradually decreased by 38% in the week when measurements were compared to those made in fed control animals. The lost intestinal mass was regained after re-feeding for 2 days in the duodenum and jejunum, and after 4 days in the ileum.

Dou and co-workers observed that morphometric measures such as wall thickness and circumference decreased during fasting. However, the thickness of the submucosal layer did not change, which may be attributed to the slow turnover rate of collagen and the short duration of the fasting period. After refeeding, the morphometric measures returned to normal, usually within 2 to 4 days. The opening angle increased in all segments after only 2 days of fasting and reached its highest value after 4 days of fasting. It then remained constant in the duodenum and ileum, but decreased in the jejunum at the end of the 7-day fasting period. The opening angle in the duodenum and jejunum was normalized after 2 days of re-feeding, and that in the ileum was normalized only after 7 days of re-feeding. It seems logical that the opening angle increases when the wall becomes softer because residual stress protects the wall against damage induced by external forces. Since fasting reduces the mucosa thickness, the compressive forces at the inner wall will be unchanged or vanish. In all segments, fasting shifted the stress-strain curves to the right. This indicates that the intestinal wall became less stiff during fasting in both circumferential and longitudinal directions. However, the change was most pronounced in the jejunum and ileum and in the longitudinal direction. This pattern of remodeling seems logical since luminal loading during fasting is greatly reduced. That is, the imposed loads from ingestion are smaller. The remodeling speed is amazingly fast considering that visible morphological change likely precedes the passive mechanical change. The change in the stress-strain properties during fasting can only partly be explained by the thinning of the wall. That is, the main thinning occurs in the epithelium, which does not by itself support much tensile stress. Re-feeding rapidly reversed the change in stress-strain.

4.6. INTERVENTIONAL EXPERIMENTAL ANIMAL MODELS

Several experiments with various kinds of intervention have been done to discover their effects on the mechanics of the intestinal wall. The studies fall into the following categories:

- Interference with the structural components of the wall (mutant mice, and enzymatic intervention),
- Pharmacologic-toxic intervention (streptozotocin-induced diabetes, and growth factor-induced remodeling),
- Surgical intervention (resection, obstruction).

Brief reports on physical intervention in the form of irradiation have also been published, but they will not be dealt with further in this book.

4.6.1. Remodeling due to Interference with the Structural Components of the Wall

In general, the structure-mechanics relationship is not well understood in the gastrointestinal wall. Despite the scarcity of data, it is generally believed that the submucosal collagen matrix is the important structural determinant of the mechanical properties of resting gastrointestinal tissue because of the high collagen content of the submucosa. In esophageal mechanics, the role of the collagen matrix is important because some diseases lead to major alterations in both collagen structure and mechanics in that organ.

4.6.1.1. Esophageal Residual Strain Properties in Mutant Mice with Osteogenesis Impefecta

The collagen matrix in the submucosa is likely the main structural determinant of the mechanical properties of resting gastrointestinal tissue because of the high collagen content of the submucosa. However, collagen fibrils are also abundant in the muscle layers where intramuscular septa are formed. The model of osteogenesis imperfecta in mutant mice (hereafter called the OIM model) as discussed in this section is important because it remodels the passive element, the collagen. Collagen is important for residual stresses, whether directly or indirectly, and also affects stresses under physiological loads. The role of the collagen matrix in esophageal mechanics is important because esophageal disease can lead to alterations in both collagen structure and esophageal mechanics. The combined results from structural and mechanical studies using the OIM mice is useful for formulation of a more precise model of the role of type I collagen fibers in esophageal mechanics. The OIM mouse exhibits many features of human osteogenesis imperfecta, such as defective skeletal development, a smaller stature, and skeletal fragility.

The OIM model was used by Gregersen *et al.* to examine the effects of type I collagen deficiency on the stress-free state of the esophagus [20]. The histological data showed that all four layers were thinner in OIM mice than in controls. The layer thickness ratio between OIM mice and controls was lower for the submucosa (0.64) than for the other layers. The average opening angle of the OIM esophagus was approximately 120° compared to approximately 90° in the control mice. Hence, a decreased amount of collagen in the esophagus of OIM mice is associated with increased residual stress. In the OIM mice, the residual strains at the surfaces of serosa and mucosa and at the interface between the mucosa-submucosa and the muscle layers were higher than in the controls. That is, the neutral axis (the plane in the wall where the tensile strain of the outer layers balances the compressive strain of the inner layers) is displaced in the mucosal direction in the OIM mice.

The data summarized above show that the most pronounced morphological and biomechanical alteration was located in the submucosa of OIM mice. As a general rule, the esophageal wall remodels itself in order to maintain optimum circumferential stresses. The high residual strain in the submucosa of the mutant mice indicates that submucosal stresses would be higher relative to those in the muscle layers during luminal loading if residual strains were non-existing. Thus, the higher residual stress and higher opening angle is needed for maintaining a uniform stress distribution. The larger residual strain in the OIM mice may affect strain gradients associated with higher strains during loading, if the tissue in the OIM mice is softer.

4.6.2. Pharmacologic-toxic Intervention

Gastrointestinal motor disorders seem to be common, both in the objectively undefined conditions (functional disease, that which is defined only in terms of symptoms) and the diseases where the cause can be determined from objective assessments of function and morphology. Some of these disorders can be imitated in animal experimental models.

One common condition that affects the gastrointestinal tract is diabetes mellitus. As many as 75% of patients visiting diabetes clinics report significant gastrointestinal symptoms. The entire gastrointestinal tract can be affected by diabetes. The common complaints include heartburn, dysphagia, early satiety, nausea, vomiting, abdominal pain, constipation and diarrhea, alone or in various combinations.

Both acute and chronic hyperglycemia can lead to specific gastrointestinal complications. Most of the gastrointestinal complications, however, seem to arise from diabetic neuropathy, the deterioration in nerve function that accompanies chronic diabetes. In the gastrointestinal tract, this represents degeneration especially of the autonomic nerves that make up the extrinsic nerves of the gut. It may also involve the intrinsic nerves, those of the enteric nervous system within the wall of the gut. As with other, mostly vascular, complications of diabetes, the long duration of the disease and a history of chronically poor glycemic control seem to be associated with more severe gastrointestinal problems. Diabetes is a disease that can be created in the laboratory and used for studying the remodeling of the mechanical properties.

4.6.2.1. Streptozotozin-Induced Diabetes

Significant remodeling of the intestine occurs in diabetes. Many histological studies have demonstrated pronounced layer proliferation during diabetes, especially the mucosa in the small intestine and esophagus. Data in rats made diabetic with a single dose of streptozotocin and studied for up to 5 weeks indicate that the small intestinal wall becomes stiffer and the opening angle and residual strain decrease in a time-dependent way after the induction of diabetes. These results are consistent with both the well-known morphological alterations in diabetes and Fung's remodeling theory. Many studies by now have been published on mechanical properties of the diabetic intestine, both in type 1 and type 2 diabetes [21-23].

4.6.2.2. Epidermal Growth Factor-Induced Remodeling

Epidermal growth factor (EGF) is a polypeptide belonging to an expanding group of growth factor ligands. The members of the EGF family, and their receptors, are widely distributed in mammals and play an important role in development, regeneration and neoplastic growth.

The whole gastrointestinal tract responds very sensitively to the effects of EGF treatment. EGF is synthesized in the salivary glands from where it is secreted in the saliva as an exocrine substance. Salivary EGF contacts the esophageal and gastric mucosa where it clearly is a factor of importance for the functional integrity of the mucosa, for mucosal protection and repair.

In the small intestine, it is well known that EGF exerts a trophic effect on the mucosa. It increases mucosal thickness and increases its surface area. Very few studies have addressed the question of the possible effects of systemic treatment with EGF on the stress-strain properties of the gastrointestinal tract or on any aspects of its biomechanical function. The results referred to below can be found in references [24-28]. Vinter-Jensen *et al.* examined the tension-strain properties of the intestinal wall after EGF treatment and found reduced circumferential wall stiffness as a result of EGF treatment. However, this study suffered from the fact that the circumferential strain was referenced to the no-load state, and the data were obtained only in the circumferential direction.

Another experiment better demonstrated EGF-induced remodeling in the small intestine. Biaxial testing (combined inflation-axial stretch) was done in rats treated with systemic EGF for up to 2 weeks, and the Kirchhoff's stress and Green's strain were computed for the circumferential and longitudinal directions. In brief, 4 constants were determined. The a_1 constant is the elastic modulus in the circumferential direction, affecting the curve for $S_{\theta\theta}$ and. $E_{\theta\theta}$. The higher a_1 , the stiffer the intestinal wall. Constant a_2 is the elastic modulus in the longitudinal direction, affecting the curve for $S_{\phi\phi}$ and $E_{\phi\phi}$. Constant a_4 is the cross modulus. Constant C fixes the scale on the stress axis.

The opening angle increased after 7 day's EGF treatment, and it continued to increase up to 14 days. In the circumferential direction, the stress-strain curves representing 4 days and 7 days of EGF treatment were shifted to the right, while the curve after 14 days of EGF treatment was shifted slightly back toward the control. In the longitudinal direction, the stress-strain curves representing 4 days and 7 days of EGF treatment were shifted to the left, but the curve after 14 days of EGF treatment was shifted back toward the control curve. Significantly smaller a_1 values were observed after 7 days and 14 days EGF treatment, and larger a_2 value were seen after 2 days and after 7 days of EGF treatment. Hence, the EGF-induced remodeling is time-dependent and the mechanical properties are anisotropic.

In the esophagus, EGF treatment also produces remodeling. The esophagus of rats treated with systemic EGF for up to 14 days has been studied *in vitro*. EGF produced wall thickening with the most pronounced effect in the mucosa. The opening angle and the absolute value of residual strains increased during the EGF treatment, indicating that more residual forces reside in the tissue during EGF treatment. The opening angle increased from approximately 110 degrees in the control animals to approximately 150 degrees after 14 days of treatment. This is consistent with the fact that the growth was more pronounced in the inner layers than in the muscle layers, in accordance with Fung's hypothesis [2]. The stress-strain curve gradually shifted to the left during the first week of EGF treatment, indicating that esophageal wall stiffness increased. The stress-strain curve shifted slightly back towards the normal state after 14 days of EGF treatment. It is likely that the non-uniform growth during EGF treatment contributes to the remodeling of the biomechanical properties. The growth of the esophagus was more pronounced during the first week, the speed of growth diminishing after 1 week of treatment. The pronounced growth of the esophagus in the first week is likely due to the direct stimulation by exogenous EGF. Endogenous EGF production may well then begin to decrease through a negative feedback mechanism. This proposed explanation may also be used to explain the similar results of another EGF experiment on the ileum by Vinter-Jensen and co-workers.

It was found that, in the normal rat esophagus, the mucosa-submucosa layer is stiffer than the muscle layer and that the stress value in the mucosa-submucosa layer is higher than it is in the muscle layer under the same loading conditions {10}. Therefore, the esophageal wall might become stiffer after EGF treatment because the mucosa-submucosa achieves more growth than the muscle layer.

4.6.3. Surgical Interventions

Models have been developed for the study of the morphometric and biomechanical remodeling after gastrointestinal obstruction and resection. Organs such as the esophagus, small intestine and the common bile duct have been partially or completely obstructed in such experiments.

4.6.3.1. Obstruction Models

Esophagus. Numerous morphometric studies have been made in the esophagus of various species, in particular in the American opossum. Placing a loose band around the distal part of the esophagus during surgery creates a partial obstruction. Schulze-Delrieu and co-workers published a series of papers primarily on the morphometric (structural) remodeling of the tissue [29-31]. Other studies found an association between the degree of dilation and the collagen content, a result that point in the direction of strain-dependent remodeling behavior. This subject obviously needs much more study to explore the mechanical changes.

The Small Intestine. Acute and chronic small bowel obstruction is a frequent clinical problem associated with high rates of morbidity and mortality. It has been estimated that 5 percent of all general surgical admissions and 20 percent of emergency surgical admissions stem from small intestinal obstruction. The long standing non-occluding obstruction of the small intestine results in tissue remodeling (morphological changes) with dilatation, wall thickening, increased collagen content, enlargement of enteric neurons, and hypertrophy of the muscular coat proximal to the site of obstruction. These changes are secondary to the accumulation of large amounts of luminal contents rostral to the obstruction, resulting in increased loading forces and deformation of the intestine. Abnormal motility occurs rostral to the obstruction with contractions of altered amplitude, frequency and duration. The studies of small intestinal obstruction discussed below were conducted before anyone in the gastroenterology was aware of the large residual strains in the small intestine. The stress-strain curves obtained, however, may be valid because recent studies have shown that the midwall strain curves does not change much if the no-load state is used as reference rather than the zeros-tress state. This assumption, however, needs to be validated in tissues affected experimentally by obstruction. Also, valid data from human subjects with obstruction are still necessary.

Partial obstruction has been created, as was done in the esophagus, by placing a loose band around the intestine [32-37]. The intestinal wall underwent massive hypertrophy proximal to the site of such a partial obstruction and dilated over the course of time. Hence, the luminal cross-sectional area and the wall thickness of the proximal segments increased in a time-dependent manner proximal to the obstruction site. The spontaneous motility in the obstructed segments consisted of irregular phasic contractions with high amplitudes (approximately 125 cmH_2O) proximal to the site of obstruction (compared to approximately 50 cmH_2O in the control animals). The disturbed motility observed after obstruction cannot necessarily be explained merely by altered properties of the muscle. The propagation time was significantly increased rostral to the obstruction site, which suggests some neurological involvement. This is consistent with Gabella's finding of disruption of the micro-anatomy of the intramural nerve plexuses in the small intestine during chronic obstruction [38, 39]. Due to thickening of the muscle layers, it was expected that the motility index would increase rostral to the obstruction site. Since a more pronounced motor response was induced in the obstructed animals than in controls, it is evident that the peristaltic reflex pathway is more sensitive to distension after obstruction than normal.

The circumferential stress-strain curves from rostral segments in the four-and two-week intervention groups of animals with partial intestinal obstruction showed a left-shifted compared to those of the distal segments of the same groups, and with the controls, indicating increased wall stiffness in the segments rostral to the obstruction. The collagen content increased in a time-dependent manner rostral to the site of obstruction. The amount, distribution, organization and kinds of collagen present in the extracellular matrix determine organ function and morphology to a large extent. A derangement in one or more of these characteristics of the collagen matrix may well cause significant structural and functional disturbances in the organ. A statistically significant association was found at the rostral location between the collagen content and the elastic modulus at a stress level of 70 kPa, indicating that collagen determines the mechanical properties in the intestine at high stress levels.

The Common Bile Duct. Biliary obstruction is a common clinical problem that may arise from neoplasm in the wall, cholelithiasis, or the compression of the lumen by external structures. However, gallstones account for most obstructions. 20% of all men and 35% of all women have gallstones by the age of 75 years. 10-15% of the stones migrate to the common bile duct and give rise to such symptoms as nausea, vomiting and pain in the right upper abdomen or epigastrium. Persistent obstruction leads to prestenotic dilatation of the common bile duct and an increase in the thickness of its wall. Several clinical and experimental studies describe the functional and anatomical changes in the obstructed common bile duct.

The most extensive work studying partial biliary obstruction from a mechanical point of view is that published by Duch *et al.* [40]. The common bile duct can be completely obstructed in pigs without their showing much evidence of secondary liver disease. The pressure in the common bile duct increased from normal values of 0.7 kPa in the control animals to approximately 3 kPa after 32 days of obstruction. The diameter and wall thickness of the common bile duct increased about three-fold at the end of the 32 days. The circumferential stress-strain relationship shifted to the right, indicating softening, in the groups studied after 3 hours, 12 hours, and 2 days, and it shifted to the left indicating stiffening, in the groups studied after 8 days and 32 days, as compared to the sham group. The longitudinal stress-strain curves were also shifted to the left of the circumferential stress-strain curves in the latter study groups, indicating a higher stiffness in the longitudinal direction. Duch *et al.* also studied the effect of reopening of the obstructed bile duct [41].

4.6.3.2. Remodeling Caused by Small Bowel Resection

The short-bowel syndrome is a difficult clinical problem, resulting from massive intestinal resection. Clinical treatments could be improved by an increased level of understanding of the physiology of the intestinal adaptation to resection. In 1888 Senn was probably the first to demonstrate intestinal remnants ability to undergo structural and functional adaptation (remodeling) in response to intestinal resection [42]. Over the last several decades, extensive animal experimentation has demonstrated a huge adaptive remodeling process in the remnant intestine after massive bowel resection. Increased villus height and crypt depth characterize the remodeling as a result of accelerated epithelial cell proliferation, smooth muscle cell hypertrophy. Dilatation and elongation of the remnant bowel also occur, leading to a greater absorptive surface area and to a prolonged transit and mucosal exposure to intra-luminal nutrition.

The extent of the remodeling depends on the resection degree and location. Dou *et al.* studied the effect of the resection of 67% of the intestine on the remodeling of the remnant intestine in rats up to four weeks after the resection [43]. The biomechanical properties were studied in terms of residual strains and stresses, and stress-strain relations with reference to the zero-stress state. The weight of the resected animals was less than the controls. The intestinal length and diameter increased more in the resected groups compared to the control groups, which resulted in a larger absorptive area. The time-dependent changes were most prominent in the ileum. Resection induced gross morphometric changes and histological remodeling characterized by proliferative increases in the wall layers. The opening angle along with the residual strain at the mucosal and serosal surfaces increased in the remnant small intestine. All changes increased as function of postoperative time and were prominent in the remnant ileum of the resected animals. The increased residual stress and residual strain may optimize the mechanical function of the remnant intestine under altered loading condition in the remnant intestine after resection.

The stress-strain relationship did not change significantly after bowel resection. Thus, the stiffness of the remnant intestine does not change for up to 4 weeks after the resection, at least, although there is clear-cut hypertrophic remodeling in the intestinal wall layers. A rapid change in the zero-stress state may have contributed to preserve stiffness during the study time. The lack of change in the stress-strain relation in remodeling after intestinal resection is consistent with the hypothesis that soft tissue remodel to maintain a uniform stress level under various conditions. The remodeling after resection seems to be directed by the requirement for a larger absorptive surface area rather than for a change in the mechanical stress and strain. The observed change in the opening angle and in the residual strain can be regarded both a result of the remodeling primarily taking place in the mucosa layer, and as a compensatory mechanism to maintain a uniform stress level.

4.7. ACTIVE MECHANICAL PROPERTIES

Chapter 1 presents the fact that the gastrointestinal tract generates the forces that produce flows in the luminal contents by three layers of muscle, one in the mucosa and two layers in the tunica muscularis. The visceral muscle cells in all three layers, roughly 100-200 microns long and 5 microns wide, are bound together roughly in parallel by a matrix of collagen fibers. The cell orientation in the muscle tissue determines the force vector generated by contractions of those cells and establishes the terminology of these muscle layers. A stroma or collagen framework confines the cells in visceral muscle, binding them into bundles that converge, diverge, and reconverge to constitute the gross muscle mass. Strong mechanical bonds tie the muscle cells to the collagen fibers in the stroma and to one another. Hence the whole structure forms a single mechanical unit.

The muscle cells lie parallel with the thick central part of one cell adjacent to the thinner extremities of others. Adjacent cells are in contact through mechanical linkages. Fibers of actin and myosin function within the cells through a sliding filament mechanism grossly similar to that skeletal muscle. The globular head of the myosin molecule interacts with the actin molecule in a cross-bridge formation. Fibers of the desmin protein organize the cell interior and transmit the forces created by the interactions of the contractile filaments to the cell membrane. These fibers converge at points on the cell membrane and at intersections within the cytoplasm. These fix the different kinds of filaments to one another and to the cell membrane. Other fine structures and elements in the smooth muscle cell that are concerned with metabolism and the cell's regulation of its own contraction are treated in Chapter 1.

It is a common fallacy to think that all aspects of gastrointestinal motor function represent the effects of nerves acting on an intrinsically passive musculature. In fact, the special properties of the visceral muscle itself determine many aspects of gastrointestinal motility. That is, the controls of contractions lie to a considerable extent in the muscle itself, and it is misleading to believe that all control is exerted by or through the innervation of the muscle.

These myogenic factors bear especially upon two matters, the rhythmicity of phasic contractions, those with a rapid onset and offset lasting only for seconds, and capacity of the muscle to generate tone, a sustained contraction. Phasic contraction has been subject of numerous studies whereas tone has received much less attention due to both methodological and conceptual difficulties.

4.7.1. Phasic Contractility

Phasic contractions have well defined beginnings and endings and last only a duration of a few seconds. They occur in all parts of the gastrointestinal tract except for the gastrointestinal sphincters and the gastric fundus. The amplitude and duration of phasic contractions vary from one part of the gut to another. For example, contractions of the esophagus and antrum often have amplitudes three-fold greater than those of the small intestine. Phasic contractions may propagate in an aboral direction (antegrade peristalsis) or in oral direction (retrograde peristalsis), or they may be stationary, not moving along the tubular conduit.

4.7.1.1. Spatial and Temporal Characteristics of Phasic Activity

Motility can be defined according to temporal properties such as to the timing of contractions with features like the duration, number, and frequency of slow waves, spikes, and contractions or contraction clusters. Thus, "temporal control" refers to the control of contractions at a given site in time. In addition motility can be characterized according to spatial properties such as to characteristics as location, direction and motion, distance and rate of spread of contractions or clusters of contractions. Hence, spatial control involves also the temporal relationship between contractions at adjacent sites.

The spatial and temporal contraction characteristics are largely responsible for the mixing and propulsion of intestinal intraluminal contents. Propulsion must be more effective when contractions occur sequentially at adjacent sites (that is, in peristalsis) than when they occur only as localized stationary events at separate loci. Other features that describe contractions are force, amplitude in space (whether the contractions are occluding or non-occluding), duration and shape (whether they are concentric or eccentric, symmetrical or asymmetrical, in both axial and circumferential directions).

Both the spatial and temporal properties of contractions are critically dependent on the electrical properties of the muscle layers, especially the frequency and propagation velocity of the electrical slow waves that constitute the basic electrical rhythm in some but not all parts of the gut. Of course, nerves and chemical or hormonal factors constitute a part of the control system as well. The interactions, in the motions of gastrointestinal tract, of nerves, hormones, and the intrinsic properties of the muscle poses as great a challenge to understanding as any that exists in physiology.

Various contractile and motor patterns of the gastrointestinal tract have been described and several terms are used to denote them. The contractile patterns describe specific patterns of activity, such as parts of what is called the migrating motor complex (MMC).

It is beyond the scope of this book to give a detailed description of the contractile patterns in all the organs of the gastrointestinal tract. The patterns vary considerable from organ to organ and change under changing conditions in each organ. The fluid mechanical consequences of these various patterns have not been described in detail.

4.7.1.2. Origin of Rhythmicity and Slow Waves

The regions of the gut that exhibit rhythmic contractions also display a rhythmic electrical phenomenon called the basic electrical rhythm, which constitutes the generation of pace making signals, the electrical slow waves. Those parts of the gastrointestinal tract that do not generate phasic contractions lack such signals. Intracellular microelectrode recordings from smooth muscle cells in rhythmically active gut parts show electrical slow waves as a signal with a rapid depolarization, a plateau, and a slower repolarization. Spike bursts are a group of very rapid transients on the plateau of the slow wave. The slow waves represent rhythmic fluctuations in the transmembrane potential of the muscle cells, coordinated in time and space throughout the muscle mass by way of electrical connections between adjacent cells. These fluctuations reflect the ionic movements through interacting ion channels in the membrane. The ion-specific channels can open or close to pass potassium, calcium, and perhaps other ions, interacting to create the consistent slow fluctuation in transmembrane potential that constitutes the electrical slow wave. That is, the different ion channels in the muscle cell membrane open and close in response to changes in the intracellular milieu that result from the action of them all together. This complex subject lies outside the scope of this book. The interactions among these channels also accounts for the generation of spikes, the action potentials that signal the initiation of a phasic contraction, as well as the slow waves.

The interstitial cells of Cajal, in relation to which the slow waves are now believed to originate, are so similar to and closely related to muscle cells as to be considered as a subtype of muscle, perhaps specially adapted to the support of the pacemaker function of the muscle.

4.7.1.3. Synapses and Neural Circuits

Nerves affect other tissues through specialized points for communication between nerve cells and other kinds of cells called synapses. Such communication involves especially the spread of a chemical substance from the nerve cell to the receiving cell. Structures in both the nerve cell and the receiving cell at these points exhibit morphological, physiological and biochemical specializations related to the sequence of events that occur in synaptic transmission. These events involve the synthesis, storage, release, diffusion, binding, and degradation or utilization of the neurotransmitter substances.

Neurotransmitters are stored in the vesicles within presynaptic axonal varicosities and are synthesized there by special biochemical systems. The arrival of the axonal nerve impulse activates the influx of calcium ions, thereby rupturing the vesicles to release the stored neurotransmitter, which then diffuses across the synaptic gap. Some of the neurotransmitter encounters receptors, chemospecific sites on the postsynaptic membrane, where it acts to initiate electrical transients in the postsynaptic membrane. The released transmitter is simultaneously removed by chemospecific enzymes from the synaptic cleft.

This brief outline describes transmission by the two best-studied neurotransmitters of the myenteric plexus, acetylcholine and noradrenaline. Other substances identified in the myenteric plexus as neurotransmitters include a variety of amino acids and small peptides, which all are larger molecules than noradrenaline and acetylcholine, and the nitric oxide gas. Although the role of all such neurotransmitter substances in principle must involve the same basic processes (synthesis, storage, release, diffusion, binding, and degradation), these other neurotransmitters likely differ from acetylcholine and noradrenaline in many aspects. For example, nerve terminals seems not suited for storage of unstable and highly diffusible gas such as nitric oxide. This gas must be synthesized on demand and diffuse into the synaptic space. For most neurotransmitters most of these neurotransmission steps remain to be described in detail.

Neuromuscular synapses in gastrointestinal muscle are diffuse; an axon branches to spread widely throughout the muscle mass, contacting thousands of cells muscle cells. In this way its transmitter affects a large body of the muscle when it is released from the varicosities. Also, the domains of separate axons from different nerve cells overlap very extensively, so one muscle cell may lie under the control of more than one nerve cell. In other words, there is no possibility for a fixed ratio of nerve cells to muscle cells in the visceral muscle of the gut as there is in somatic muscle.

Bioengineering has made essentially no contribution to our understanding of the process of synaptic transmission or to the effect of the geometry of the nerves in visceral muscle on the behavior of that muscle. Still, such physical processes as diffusion are involved, and engineering principles may have much to contribute to our understanding of these matters.

4.7.1.4. How the Gut Induces Different Motor Patterns

The enteric nervous system has a major place in the neural control of intestinal motor patterns. Basic circuits serve as the pathways for the peristaltic reflex, in which mechanical stimulation of the gut at a point induces contractions rostral to the point of stimulation and inhibition caudal to that point.

The idea that this reflex fully accounts for peristalsis throughout the gut is clearly unacceptable, in spite of the fact that it is widely viewed as having that responsibility. For one thing, the reflex does not seem to be present in the esophagus, stomach or colon. For another, if it were the only mechanism in the small intestine, flow through the intestine would be much faster than it is. For another thing, the reflex in the intestine appears to be an on-off phenomenon, a fact that makes it difficult to reconcile with the clearly regulated and varying quantitative aspects of gastrointestinal contractions and flow.

The likelihood is that the reflex is oriented as it is simply because, if a mechanoreceptive reflex must be present, it must, on teleological grounds, be so arranged to be consistent with the polarity that the intestine manifests in so many other respects.

We cannot view rationally the enteric nervous control of the gut as an intricate computer-like network of reflex pathways bringing about, through programming, the complex spatiotemporal events involved in motility. It seems more a matter of equilibrium between excitatory and inhibitory elements that simultaneously bear upon the mechanical apparatus. The muscle responds continuously to the nerves, its response reflecting the summation of the two opposite influences. The muscle can respond to neural activation only as the slow waves pass along the gut, for they establish the series of brief intervals when the muscle is able to respond to neural excitation. Thus, the slow waves determine the frequency and the propagation velocity of intestinal contractions. The nerves establish the likelihood of contraction as a continuously variable function.

Stationary circumferential contractions, producing the pattern called segmentation, might be produced by a brief excitation of a short intestinal segment. If a slow wave passes over this short segment, spike potentials are induced and a local contraction occurs. Propagated contraction waves, peristalsis, might be produced by brief excitations of long intestinal segments. The slow wave, which moves over the excited segment, will induce spikes and produces a contraction because excitatory nerves over a long segment are activated simultaneously. This kind of excitation occurs irregularly in space and time; consequently, the contraction waves start at variable loci and spread over variable distances of the gut. Clusters of contractions might be produced by the prolonged excitation of a short intestinal segment. When consecutive slow waves move over the excited segment synaptic rhythmic but spatially localized peristaltic contractions are produced. When the prolonged excitation remains at the same locus, a stationary cluster occurs. When the segment of excitation migrates a migrating cluster is produced.

4.7.1.5. Bolus Transport Mechanics

Flow and bolus transport in distensible organs such as the gastrointestinal tract are influenced by many factors. The driving forces are the pressure generated by the peristaltic contractions and, to a minor extent, hydrostatic force including that of gravity. Brasseur and co-workers demonstrated that bolus volume, viscosity and abdominal compression influence bolus pressure in the esophagus [44, 45]. Factors like the shape and size of the luminal cross-section, and the tissue viscoelastic properties like the elastic modulus and shear modulus of the wall are also important determinants of flow, as predicted by biomechanical models. Studies in guinea-pigs and pigs have shown that differences in luminal cross-sectional area and passive elastic properties exist between proximal and distal regions in the esophagus and small intestine, and the passive stress-strain properties are now well described. Such findings are associated with the well-known differences in flow properties and motility between these regions. Brasseur demonstrated that the bolus pressures in the human esophagus range up to 3-5 kPa. Hence, the bolus pressure corresponds to the most elastic part of the distension curves, a mechanism that reduces resistance to flow.

Gastrointestinal distensibility studies may help us understand the complex fluid mechanical behavior in the tract. Thus far, flow properties in the esophagus have been studied by Brasseur *et al.* [44, 45] while primarily Christensen's group described gastric emptying, antroduodenal mechanics, and intestinal flow properties [46, 47]. Ehrlein's group, Meyer and co-workers, Schulze-Delrieu and co-workers as well as by a few other investigators. Mathematical modeling of peristaltic transport in distensible tubes has been published by Stavitsky, Fung, and Miftakhov [7, 47-49] among others. The modeling of peristaltic transport is based on the premise that the interaction between bolus transport and gastrointestinal elasticity is best understood by examining the fluid dynamics equations and equations describing gastrointestinal deformation and stresses (the constitutive equations). The boundary conditions govern the interaction between these equations.

4.7.1.6. Intestinal Reflexes and Mechanoreceptors

Peristalsis is the coordinated movement of alimentary muscle resulting in the propulsion of intraluminal contents. The intestinal mechanisms controlling peristalsis are contained within the enteric wall, so that propulsive motility can be studied *in vitro*. Trendelenburg was the first, in 1917, to describe an *in vitro* method for studying peristalsis, using guinea-pig ileum [50]. By raising the intraluminal pressure in a segments of intestine mounted in an organ bath, he was able to make it dilate until a sudden contraction of the longitudinal layer followed by a propagated contraction of the circular muscle emptied its contents. Trendelenburg distinguished between a preparatory phase and an emptying phase in this reflex. By use of different modifications of the Trendelenburg method, it was demonstrated that the two phases had little in common except for being elicited by the same stimulus. This stimulus is circumferential stretching rather than increased transmural pressure. The two phases of the response are differently regulated and the phases are influenced by a large number of pharmacological and bioactive substances as might be expected of nerve-mediated responses.

Fig. (**7**) shows an example of distension-induced contractility in the human esophagus. Such reflexes are initiated either by distension of the intestinal wall by a balloon or by the intraluminal instillation of liquid for the chemical stimulation of the mucosa through the excitation of chemoreceptors.

Since balloon distension elicits a reflex, mechanoreceptors must exist in the neural elements in the sensory nerve terminals of the gastrointestinal wall. Many physiologists assume or believe that the receptors are pressure-sensitive or volume-sensitive. However, mechanoreceptors in the gut are not directly sensitive to variations in pressure or volume. A large variation in the pressure and volume thresholds needed to trigger the peristaltic reflex has been found in various studies and species, indicating that pressure is not the direct stimulus. Instead, the receptors are stimulated by forces and deformations in the intestinal wall that can arise from changes in transmural pressure through stretch of the wall. The same mechanism accounts for the operation of baroreceptors in the cardiovascular system. Despite the name (baro means pressure), the baroreceptor nerve activity is associated with wall deformation rather than with pressure, because restricting wall movement abolishes baroreceptor-mediated reflexes. It has been shown in a similar fashion that stretch is the potent and direct stimulus of gastrointestinal mechanoreceptors rather than increased transmural pressure. Since the receptors are also stimulated by visceral tension and deformation developed during intestinal contractions further suggests that they are sensitive to deformation.

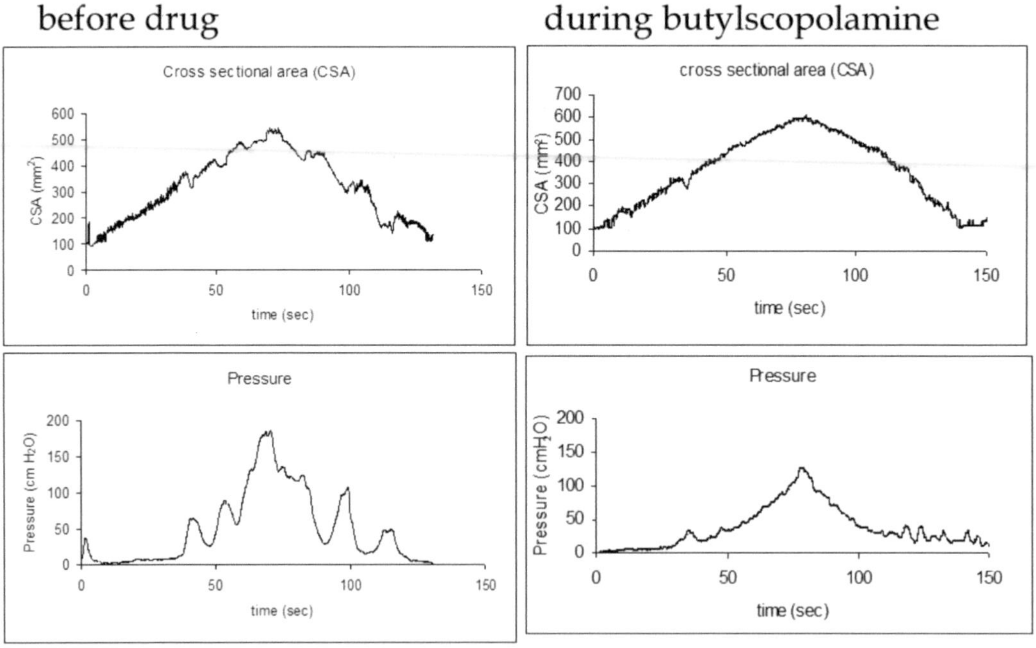

Figure 7: Illustration of esophageal cross-sectional area (CSA) and pressure during bag distension before and during the administration of butylscopolamine.

Since pressure is not the direct stimulus, but the indirect one, a large error is likely to arise when the receptor response is expressed as a function of pressure. Such an approach makes it impossible to draw useful conclusions from investigations where pressure is quantified as though it is the direct mechanoreceptive stimulus. Further analysis must consider the fact that the mechanical forces imposed on the tissue by balloon inflation induce stresses and strains in various directions. Thus, distension must cause both longitudinal tensile stress and strain and radial compressive stress and strain in addition to circumferential tensile stress and strain. For the study of mechanoreceptor kinematics, it is therefore important to express the stimulus in terms of magnitude and direction of the stress, strain, and strain rate. It is not possible to measure strains and stresses exactly at the receptor sites. Theoretical solutions based on experimentally-determined mechanical properties in different layers of the gastrointestinal wall may therefore be necessary in a numerical analysis. By determining the nature of these mechanical stimuli we may learn more about the mechanoreceptors and how they adapt to the physical environment. This will allow us to establish the relation between the activity in the neurons, the electrical responses of neurons, and the mechanical behavior of the gut. On the other hand, if the appropriate mechanical stimulus is not known, the data are merely qualitative. Models that preserve the structural integrity of the tissue to most closely reproduce the physical condition of the organ *in vivo* are most useful in this respect.

4.7.2. Gastrointestinal Smooth Muscle Tone

This subject is reviewed in detail in Gregersen and Christensen [51], from which the sections below is a summary. In the biomedical world, the stable resistance to stretch that characterizes tissues containing muscle is designated as tone. Both the fixed physical properties of the tissue (passive resistance) and the energy-consuming activation of the contractile apparatus of the muscle (active resistance) contribute to the resistance.

Somatic muscle contracts when stretched. The absence of such contraction, loss of tone, signifies neurological disease. For many physicians and physiologists, tone refers only to the active resistance to stretch arising from muscle contraction. Therefore, terms as "passive tone" and "active tone" are confusing and unnecessary because other terms make the distinction between passive and active mechanical properties. By definition tone is active.

Tone also occurs in visceral muscle. The notion of muscle tone is essential in gastrointestinal physiology. Tone in gut muscle, as compared to that in striated muscle, has until recent decades received little attention when the significance in the gastrointestinal motility became evident. Tone affects the fundamental diameter of the gastrointestinal conduit. For this reason a crucial property of gastrointestinal muscle is the capacity to generate tone, especially in gastrointestinal sphincters and in the parts that serve reservoir functions allowing pooling to occur. Such parts are the gastric fundus, the terminal ileum, the cecum and colon. Studies of tone must take into account the science of biomechanics as well as those of physiology and anatomy.

4.7.2.1. Myogenic Tone and Neurogenic Tone

Tone generated in somatic muscle is neurogenic by nature. It represents a constant low level of discharge of the excitatory innervation. In contrast, some tone in the gut is a property of the muscle itself rather than being generated by the constant discharge of excitatory nerves. In gastrointestinal sphincters the muscle exhibits myogenic tone. This is evidenced since some part of the resistance to stretch is unaffected by tetrodotoxin and blockers of synaptic transmission. Not all tone in the gut is myogenic, however. Excitatory nerves and hormones also affect the contraction force in sphincters and elsewhere. Some evidence exist that sphincter muscle is more sensitive to excitatory drugs than non-sphincter muscle. The same properties that are responsible for myogenic tone may enhance its sensitivity to hormones and to drugs that act through autonomic receptor mechanisms.

Tone is contrasted to phasic contraction based on the temporal characteristics of the two kinds of contraction. The distinct temporal differences between the two forms of contractile behavior show the need for precise criteria to distinguish them quantitatively. The time between the contraction onset and offset is measurable in terms of seconds with only slight variability. Such events recur at a reasonably constant frequency at any particular location. In contrast, the duration of the tonic contractions can be measured in minutes or hours. Furthermore, tonic contractions show no obvious pattern or regularity in occurrence.

Tonic contractions may arise in two different ways. Mandrek and Golenhofen postulated a dual origin for tone based on studies on isolated intestinal muscle strips [52]. Evidence was provided for two different contractile mechanisms producing, respectively, tonic and phasic (or rhythmic) contractions and they pointed out the existence of two types of tone (Fig. **8**). "Tetanic tone" represents fused phasic (or rhythmic) contractions at one locus as they pointed out. Tetanic tone represents rhythmic contractions of a sufficient high frequency and force that do not allow sufficient time for the repeating contractile onsets and offsets to be apparent. The second type was named "specific tone" that was characterized as a sustained contraction at one locus. Whereas specific tone appears to be fundamentally myogenic, tetanic tone seems likely to be at least partly neurogenic.

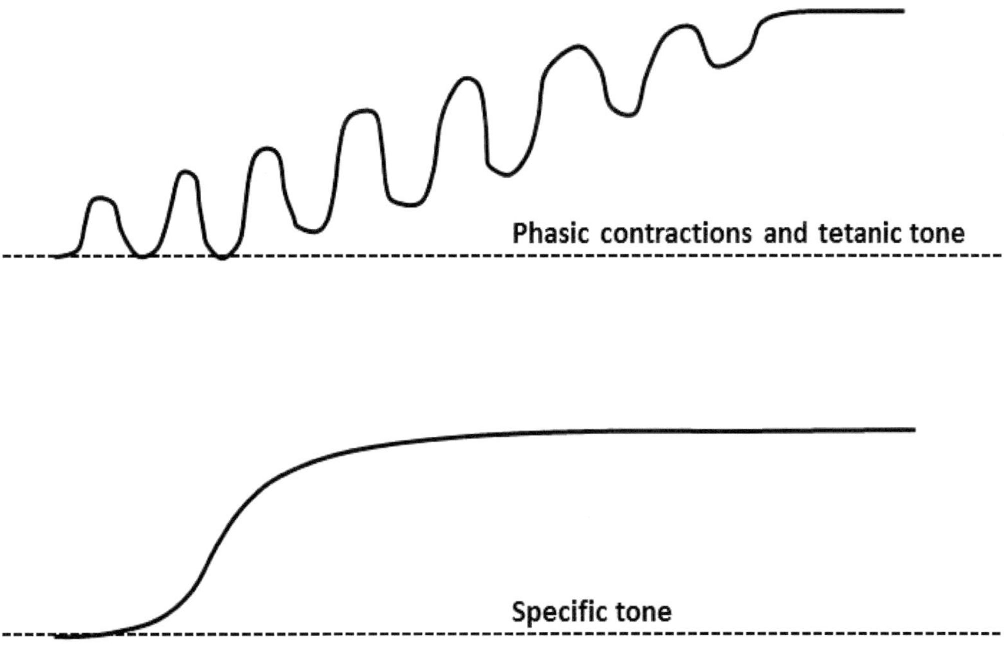

Figure 8: Diagram showing tetanic and specific tone.

Mandrek and Golenhofen demonstrated that the two types of tone could be distinguished experimentally [52]. Muscle cells involved in phasic contractions generate slow waves which are slow changes in membrane potential. Phasic contractions arise when the contraction machinery is activated which occur by a Ca^{++} influx usually associated with spike potentials. Therefore, the tonic contractions of tetanic nature may be associated with the presence of slow waves and spikes. Absence of slow waves and spikes indicates the presence of specific or myogenic tone.

Mandrek and Golenhofen also suggested that specific tone and tetanic tone could be distinguished on pharmacological grounds. The calcium channel antagonist nifedipine abolishes phasic contractions whereas tonic contractions in general remain unaltered or only respond to higher concentrations of such agents. Nifedipine can suppress tetanic tone completely since tetanic tone is controlled by spike discharges resulting in phasic contractions that fuse together. Specific tone is preferentially suppresses by sodium nitroprusside, by activating guanylate synthase according to Mandrek and Golenhofen.

4.7.2.2. Evidence for Tone In Vivo

The demonstration of tone *in vitro* in gastrointestinal muscle strips is relatively straightforward but the measurement of tone *in vivo* is not. The conventional manometry as done in many laboratories to record gastrointestinal motor function cannot detect tone in the intact gastrointestinal tract except in sphincteric regions. Even in sphincters, the recorded pressures cannot be regarded as linear reflections of the degree of tone. Still, many investigators seem to accept the sphincter pressure recorded by conventional manometric techniques or the volume of a non-sphincteric region at a constant pressure as faithful representations of tone. They approach is not correct. Such changes may be caused or influenced by several factors. A critical look at the evidence for tone, especially in non-sphincteric regions, is necessary before drawing clear-cut conclusions about the nature of tone in the various gastrointestinal segments.

Tone in Sphincters. Gastrointestinal sphincters are specialized regions with sustained muscle contraction. For example tonic contraction in the lower esophageal sphincter normally generates a sustained intraluminal pressure of about 30 mmHg. This is apparently specific tone because this sphincter normally exhibits no rhythmicity. In addition, the tone is not related to slow wave or spike activity. In the manometric definition of sphincters, the pressure represents the resistance to the flow of water through the side hole of the perfused tube or the force on a solid state transducer. The flow resistance or force is the result of the approximation of the wall of the esophagus to the catheter. The quantification of tone measured in this way is unacceptable as anything more than a distorted reflection. Both because manometrically recorded pressure is not linearly related to the contraction force and because several passive factors enter into the measurement. Such passive factors include the physical properties and geometry of the mucosa, the geometry of the sphincter and the tethering of the esophagus to external structures in the diaphragmatic hiatus. A short sleeve mounted over the catheter tip, basically converting it to a balloon, give more consistent results in measuring sphincteric tone. However, it simply integrates or averages the passive and active factors rather than eliminating the passive factors, and the relationship between tone and manometric pressure is still not linear.

The demonstration of myogenic tone in the lower esophageal sphincter immediately adjacent to muscle devoid of such tone in the esophageal body makes the comparison of the two kinds of muscle obvious. Apparently there is a greater proportion of collagen in the sphincter. However, it has not been demonstrated that the excess collagen correlates with a greater passive resistance to stretch. The muscle itself in the lower esophageal sphincter seems to differ from the muscle of the esophageal body. The sphincter muscle seems to have mitochondria that occupy a greater fraction of space in the muscle and the mitochondria tend to be more centrally located in the cells. Furthermore, the myogenic tone is oxygen dependent in the sphincter. In contrast, the phasic contractions of the esophageal body are not. In addition more cytochrome C activity is a feature of sphincteric muscle. All the above points to a distinction in energy production when generating myogenic tone. Studies by Szymanski suggest differences in contractile proteins and the calcium-binding proteins [53]. Thus, the literature on the lower esophageal sphincter seems to confirm the hypothesis that specific tone is myogenic. Hence it reflects the activity of a different kind of muscle from that which generates rhythmic contractions.

Christensen and Torres long ago demonstrated myogenic tone in the oblique muscle layer of the stomach in contrast to that found in the other two layers [54], and it seems superficially at least to be indistinguishable from that of the lower esophageal sphincter. In fact, the two muscle structures seem to be anatomically continuous, where the sphincter appears to be a part of the gastric sling fibers that constitute the edge of the oblique muscle layer. It seems feasible that a specific set of characteristics of gastrointestinal muscle establishes it as tonic muscle. The same features may in the same way be found expressed in a greater or lesser degree in tonic muscle in other gastrointestinal sphincters such as the pylorus or internal anal sphincter.

The pyloric sphincter and the ileocecal sphincter also express tone, though little has been done to try to measure it *in vivo*. The internal anal sphincter also expresses tone. Indeed the basic properties of the muscle in the internal anal sphincter closely resemble those of the lower esophageal sphincter.

The persisting belief that some distinction in enteric nerve function characterizes the tonic sphincteric regions of the gastrointestinal tract may be accounted for by the evidence of greater sensitivity to autonomic drugs acting through membrane receptors in the lower esophageal sphincter. The same special features that generate tonic contraction in the muscle also seem to increase the responsiveness to excitatory neurohormones. This sort of evidence has not been looked for in other sphincteric regions. It would not be surprising if this property were found to characterize specific tone in general.

Tone in Non-sphincteric Regions. Tonic contractions can also be generated by smooth muscle outside sphincteric regions. Such tone is more difficult to detect than tone in sphincters. Tonic contractions can occur without measuring an elevation of baseline pressure even at the same time that short-lasting phasic contractions may be recorded. This can occur because the small intraluminal pressure caused by the tonic muscle contraction is reasonably stable. Another reason is that the pressure dissipates into regions adjacent to the site of the recording when nothing confines it. This is now usually termed the "common-cavity" phenomenon. For such reasons, in most of the gastrointestinal tract tone cannot be detected by means of ordinary manometry. Detection of tonic contractions of this type requires a distending balloon that confines the pressures allowing them to be recorded.

Tone is a major feature of the gastric fundus where extensive work has been done. Gastric relaxation mediated by nonadrenergic noncholinergic inhibitory nerves has a significant role in establishing the reservoir function of this part of the stomach. Receptive relaxation is related to expansion of the fundus, occurring from a constricted state that represents the tonic contraction mainly in the oblique muscle layer. This is maintained in the absence of slow waves and spike activity. Hence the tone seems to be specific tone which is confirmed by the fact that this muscle exhibits myogenic tone *in vitro*. Gastric tone is measured *in vivo* more or less exclusively by the volume variations in an intragastric balloon with a constant low intraluminal pressure. This is the so-called barostat technique but it has many limitations (see below and in chapter 2).

Good evidence for tone in the small intestine is available, though the data often are qualitative by nature. The main evidence is as follows:

- The small intestine dilates in chronic intestinal pseudo-obstruction and during the administration of smooth muscle relaxants such as glucagon. This indicates that some level of basal tone exists there under normal conditions.

- Animal studies using serosal strain gauge transducers and video fluoroscopy indicate that tonic muscle contractions in the small intestine occur during the fasted state.

- Impedance planimetry has demonstrated the presence of specific tone in the human duodenum during phase I of the migrating motor complex [55]. The tone in phase I was evident as a stable reduction in the luminal cross-sectional area that increased with the onset of phase II. This is consistent with a difference in the active muscle contractile state between the two phases. The finding of tone in phase I is surprising because phase I is essentially devoid of action potentials (spikes) and contractions, whereas phase II is characterized by constant bursts of spike or action potential activity and contractions. Thus, an inverse relationship exists between spike activity (phasic contractions) and tone in phase I and in phase II of the migrating motor complex. Tone is present in phase I when spikes are absent but absent in phase II when spikes occur. This is specific tone and is a representation of the Mandrek-Golenhofen concept of dualism, demonstrating that tone and phasic contractions represent different modes of activation of the contractile apparatus.

In the colon and rectum long-lasting tonic contractions are frequently recorded. A few studies by Mayrand have also claimed the existence of tone in the esophageal body [56, 57], though it is unclear if the fluid mechanical function of the esophagus would gain anything from tone in the esophageal body. However, tone would aid buckling of the mucosa and may increase resistance to flow.

4.7.2.3. A Mechanical Definition of Tone

Tone is a mechanical phenomenon. Consequently, physiologists must deal with the mechanical stress and strain concepts. Thus, proper consideration of the tissue mechanics and geometry of the various sites and organs organ under scrutiny must be taken.

Stress is the force per unit area, and strain is a dimensionless measure of deformation, as described in chapter 2. Muscle can develop active force and thereby to contract, often in response to applied stress. Two kinds of stress are created. One kind arises from the passive tissue mechanical properties. The other kind arises from the activation of the muscle contractile apparatus in accordance with the Hill model. There are both active and passive forms of stress. The active form of stress can be both tone and phasic contractions. Considering the issue of tone in uni-axial terms, smooth muscle tone results in a sustained reduction in the specimen length under isotonic conditions. In contrast isometric conditions where strain is prevented allow the development of maximal active stress. Gastrointestinal smooth muscle operates mostly under isotonic conditions *in vivo*, allowing itself to shorten with little resistance. Hence, the amount of active stress developing in the muscle is minimized. In manometric studies and in studies with balloons, the isotonic conditions are violated to some extent. The presence of an object in the lumen that resists compression by limiting the muscle shortening magnifies the active stress developed. That is why the pressure recorded manometrically from the lower esophageal sphincter varies directly with the diameter of the recording catheter.

The gastrointestinal tract can in many parts be considered a reasonably uniform cylinder. Therefore, it makes sense in geometric terms to define tone as a sustained active stress producing strain that leads to a reduction in luminal circumference and cross-sectional area, or in surface area. The activation of the smooth muscle induces the stress. For the more irregular globular parts of the gastrointestinal tract such as the gastric fundus, the gallbladder and the cecum, it is more appropriate to view the strain as a factor tending to reduce the surface area rather than reducing the volume. The reason is the high degree of radial asymmetry in these irregular regions. Even in perfect spheres, the volume and surface area are not linearly related. Their relationship is quite problematical in an irregular globular organ like the stomach.

Most studies of tone *in vivo* define tone in terms of changes in "strain" (volume at a predefined pressure level, or a change in the slope of the volume-pressure curve (compliance curve, $\Delta V/\Delta P$). However, there is no knowledge of the nature of the active or passive stresses. Such a definition naturally leads to confusion due to the complicated relationship between stress and strain. The stress-based definition and measurement of tone rather than as strain or deformation imply the need for the knowledge of forces related to the active and the passive stress components.

The passive tissue properties that characterize living muscle may contribute a large fraction of the resistance to stretch. Therefore, it may be falsely identified as active properties contributing to tone. However, phenomena that at a glance look like tone may not actually be tone. An example is that when the esophagus is excised from the body it shortens to half its *in vivo* length. This is not a representing tone but merely the manifestation of a huge passive longitudinal stress in the esophagus *in vivo*, likely the largest found anywhere in the body even exceeding that of arteries.

4.7.2.4. Why Tone Cannot be Measured by Pressure-Volume Measurements

Significant problems exist when using pressure-volume measurements in balloons to record tone and distensibility. Many investigators are unaware of the problems they face from the obscurities of gastrointestinal physiology as well as from lack of knowledge of the mechanical principles that apply to the distension of balloon placed in the gastrointestinal tract. The problems relate to many factors such as the probe design, the measurement method, geometric considerations, balloon properties, and assumptions the analysis is based on. Actually, pressure-volume measurement in the gut cannot accurately measure tone. The bulleted paragraphs below points out some of the significant problems.

- The whole balloon surface area must be in contact with the tissue. This state is never completely attained in volume measurements in the intestine and stomach. However, efforts should be made to approach the ideal contact, otherwise the failure to achieve proper contact can lead to major error.

- It must be ensured that the applied pressure is transmitted as completely as possible to the tissue. This requires that the balloon is large for it not to contribute its own elastic properties which would affect the results of the measurements. The applied pressure must also be confined to the wall itself assuming that the surrounding structures do not contribute by their own elastic properties or by tethering.

- The hysteresis of the balloon and infusion system as well as the friction between the tissue and balloon wall must be taken into account.

- Studies making use of long balloons provide data that are difficult to interpret. The reason is that simultaneous excitation and inhibition of phasic activity is likely to occur at the proximal and distal ends of the balloon. Short balloons may encounter only few phasic contractions whereas long balloons sum up multiple phasic contractions over the balloon length to produce a stable pressure or volume that easily masquerades as tone. Volume measurements in a long balloon may consequently show little or no change when the changes in shape in the balloon are considerable.

- Any balloon will inevitable show tendency to elongate rather than to distend the organ in radial direction. The reason is that the tubular organ resists radial expansion more than the balloon material resists its expansion in the axial direction (see chapter 3, Figs. **3** and **4**). The degree of balloon elongation obviously depends on the balloon material. Very compliant latex balloons are often used in pressure-volume measurements. However, polyethylene or polyurethane bags are now used more often, but some degree of elongation inevitably occurs with any balloon. Wall tension and compliance are overestimated with balloon elongation and even a small error in calculating balloon volume in the low-pressure range will affect the results of any stress-strain analysis since the basal radius, r_0, is determined in this range in studies *in vivo* (where the true zero-stress state cannot be determined).

- A circular cross-section is assumed in pressure-volume techniques that distend balloons to study tone in tubular organs. However, studies in animals clearly show that the small intestine has an elliptical cross-section at low inflation pressures. The false assumption of a circular cross-section is not a trivial matter. The volume-to-surface area relationship in an elliptical cylinder is complex and stress exhibit a non-uniformly distribution in the circumference of an elliptical cylinder.

- Since the surface area of a globular viscus cannot be measured directly *in vivo*, investigators have used methods to measure volume is such organs with the assumption that their balloon systems can follow changes in the tone of the wall of the globe by measuring variations in volume (representing length). This is fundamentally wrong in respect to the stomach since the stomach is not spherical. The tension induced in the stomach wall by distension is not distributed uniformly because of the geometric asymmetry. Furthermore, phasic contractions moving through the distal stomach will inevitable affect the measured volume since part of the balloon will likely extends into that region. Thus, such methods to measure gastric tone yield only an approximation of tone, and the errors may be large.

- The distensibility of the gastrointestinal tract depends upon both the passive properties of the muscle and its physiological state *in vivo*. Smooth muscle cells are oriented both circumferentially and longitudinally in all the gastrointestinal organs. Furthermore, the contractile state of both layers independently must affect both the wall stiffness and the lumen geometry. Longitudinal muscle contraction increases the intestinal diameter and tends to excite circular layer contraction at the site of distension. Such factors indicate that distensibility as measured with balloons can be affected, not only by the amount of phasic contractility and tone in the circular muscle layer but also by the relative activities of the two muscle layers. To a large degree, phasic contractions in both layers can be eliminated by the administration of drugs that may have less or even little effect on myogenic tone. Yet it is difficult to access the tone and the passive properties of gastrointestinal muscle *in vivo* for the other reasons given above, quite aside from the confusion that may be created by the possibility of phasic contractions occurring simultaneously in the two major muscle layers.

- Many investigators seem not to give insufficient consideration to the experimental protocol. For example many appear to be unaware that a specific loading pressure can be reached at different volumes which are dependent on the loading history. The investigator must take into account two forms of history-dependent mechanical behavior namely the time-dependent viscoelasticity and the load-dependent strain softening in repeated distension protocols. Careful consideration must be taken regarding the reproducibility of the results in distension protocols and to design them specifically for the intended purpose.

4.7.2.5. Tone and Gastric Accommodation

Gastric accommodation is important for gastric function. It has become a key mechanism for the understanding of functional dyspepsia pathophysiology. It may well be relevant for symptom generation in other disorders. Gastric accommodation can be assessed by several methods. The barostat is considered to be the gold standard for measuring proximal gastric accommodation. With the barostat gastric tone is estimated by recording variations in the air volume inside an intragastric bag that is maintained at a constant pressure by the barostat (hence the name). The idea is that accommodation of the proximal stomach is reflected in changes of gastric tone. However, the invasive method affects normal gastric motility. The bag likely also alters intragastric distribution and emptying of the meal, the direct stimulus being imposed by the bag itself on the stomach wall. This may result in increased antral distension. For these reasons, non-invasive methods as MRI, SPECT, and ultrasonography are warranted for the study of gastric accommodation.

The gastric accommodation process has been explored as a concept for over 100 years, evaluating relaxation of the proximal stomach. Receptive relaxation was defined as a vagal reflex, aiding dilation of the corpus-fundus region of the stomach in response to swallowing, vomitation or oesophageal stimulation. Adaptive relaxation represents an intrinsic vagovagal reflex enabling the stomach to increase its volume markedly without a corresponding pressure increase. Adaptive relaxation enables the stomach to maintain a relatively low pressure and to continuously adapt the volume to its content.

The term gastric accommodation is far too complex to embrace in one definition. The reason is that it is utilized in at least 3 different meanings in the literature: These meanings are the accommodation *process*, the accommodation *reflex*, and the accommodation *response*. Furthermore, the term is common in everyday language expressing that "the stomach accommodates a meal". It was also used in 1963 by Paton and Vane to describe gastric "expansion to accommodate the fluid" [58]. Gastric accommodation is a complex phenomenon reflecting how the gastric compartment size changes in response to a meal. Both intra- and extragastric reflexes are involved. The extragastric reflexes comprise receptive relaxation as well as intestine-gastric reflexes that are elicited by balloon distension or duodenal nutrient infusion. The intragastric reflexes include adaptive relaxation and proximal stomach relaxation induced from antral reflexes.

An accommodation *reflex* has been discovered with demonstration of intragastric pressure regulated by gastric "accommodation to distension". This reflex is elicited when continuous volume expansion of the proximal stomach reaches a critical level. Hereby relaxation of smooth muscles of the gastric wall is induced in order to prevent further increase in pressure. This phenomenon is a reflex arc consisting of mechanoreceptors located in the gastrointestinal wall, neuro-muscular pathways through ENS, and a well-defined response in the effector organ. The reflex seems mediated through the vagus nerve but local axon reflexes may also be involved. The term accommodation *response* is the result of the *reflex* or the effect of the *process*. This is a precise notion for what we intend to measure with different methods.

The gastric meal accommodation *process* has two components from a biomechanical perspective. One is passive meal distension of the gastric compartments and the other is active muscle relaxation of the gastric wall. The first component should ideally be measured with imaging methods whereas the second component can be measured with the barostat. However, imaging methods at this stage do not distinguish between stomach enlargements due to meal-induced distension or due to reflex relaxation. It merely measures the total accommodated volume. Neuromuscular factors are important for gastric accommodation. Therefore, it is also a matter of evaluation of the stomach mechanical properties. In this sense the barostat merely detects the change in wall tone. However, the barostat cannot as the imaging methods provide data on the volume distribution and the normal behaviour of the gastric wall. In biomechanics it is essential to understand the organ geometry. Furthermore, it is essential to understand the forces and deformation in different directions for a better understanding of the active-passive muscle function and mechano-sensation in health and in diseases. 2D and 3D image analysis of the gastric compartments are warranted.

The widely available clinical method ultrasonography has shown applicability and validity for the study of gastric accommodation. 2D ultrasonography methods developed by several scientists from the Bergen group and other groups have been implemented for studying gastric accommodation in diseases such as functional dyspepsia and diabetes. 2D ultrasonography has also been applied to study pharmacological intervention. Another advantage with is its clinical applicability.

Few methods are capable of measuring all parameters of gastric motility simultaneously. However, several publications have demonstrated the feasibility of ultrasonography to study gastric accommodation as well as gastric emptying, gastric geometry, intragastric distribution of its contents, antral motility and antral distensibility, transpyloric flow and strain of the gastric wall. For a review of data on the stomach, the reader is referred to the ultrasound book by Ødegaard, Gilja and Gregersen [59].

Abnormalities of gastric accommodation are found in several patients groups with functional or organic disorders. Determination of gastric geometry, the mechanical forces and deformation during gastric accommodation, and the relationship between active and passive muscle function are important factors to consider in those diseases.

4.8. SENSORY RESPONSES ELICITED FROM THE GASTROINTESTINAL TRACT

Although it was previously a common belief that the internal organs were devoid of sensory nerves, the idea that sensations can arise directly from the viscera is widely accepted today. According to classical and long-accepted theory, the sensory nerves that carry information that can be expressed as a conscious sensation (pain, in the case of the gut) travel together with the sympathetic nerves, whereas the afferent (sensory) nerve that travels with the parasympathetic nerves carry information that does not reach consciousness.

Visceral pain is a common expression of visceral disease and one of the most frequent reasons for patients to seek medical attention. Much of what we know about the mechanism of pain derives from experimental studies of somatic pain, not visceral pain. Despite the fact that visceral pain is an important part of the normal sensory repertoire of animals and human beings and a prominent symptom of many disease conditions, only limited clinical research has been done in this area.

The characteristics of the mechanoreceptors of the gut have been widely addressed in neurophysiological studies in experimental animals. Most of them activate non-myelinated C-fibers or small myelinated Aδ-fibers. The mechanoreceptors are predominantly localized in the muscular layers, but the mucosa, the serosa and the mesentery are also supplied. Rapidly adapting mechanoreceptors may be located in the mucosa, whereas slowly adapting mechanoreceptors are located in the intramuscular layer.

The majority of the mechanoreceptor nerve fibers respond in both physiological (that is non-painful) and painful ranges of mechanical stimulation. An essential question is whether an extreme distension of the gut, one that maximally excites mechanoreceptors and produces pain at the same time, produces that pain through excitation of the mechanoreceptors or through the excitation of a separate set of neural receptors, nociceptors. From animal studies, we know that there are three distinct classes of nociceptors in internal organs including the small intestine. The first class has a high threshold to natural stimuli (mostly mechanical). The encoding function is evoked entirely by stimuli within the noxious range. The second class of receptors has a low threshold to natural stimuli. Third, intensity-encoding nociceptors have a stimulus-response function that spans the range of stimulation intensity from innocuous to noxious.

The mechanosensitive fibers can also be divided into different populations, phasic and tonic populations, but conflicting results regarding the localization of fibers responding to different distension speed have been found in animal and human studies. Some fibers adapt to maintained distension, whereas others do not, maintaining the same magnitude of response during prolonged distension. Many mechanosensitive fibers respond to both distension of the organ and to contraction and are considered in-series with the muscle cells. Many studies of mechanoreceptors suffer from serious methodological limitations, such as the failure to measure the stimulus in biomechanical terms that apply to the wall.

Fig. (**9**) shows an example of repeated distensions in the esophagus of a healthy volunteers and a patient with non-cardiac chest pain. The healthy volunteer without problems can have ten distensions done in the esophagus up to the pain threshold whereas the patients only can take four distensions before it becomes to unpleasant.

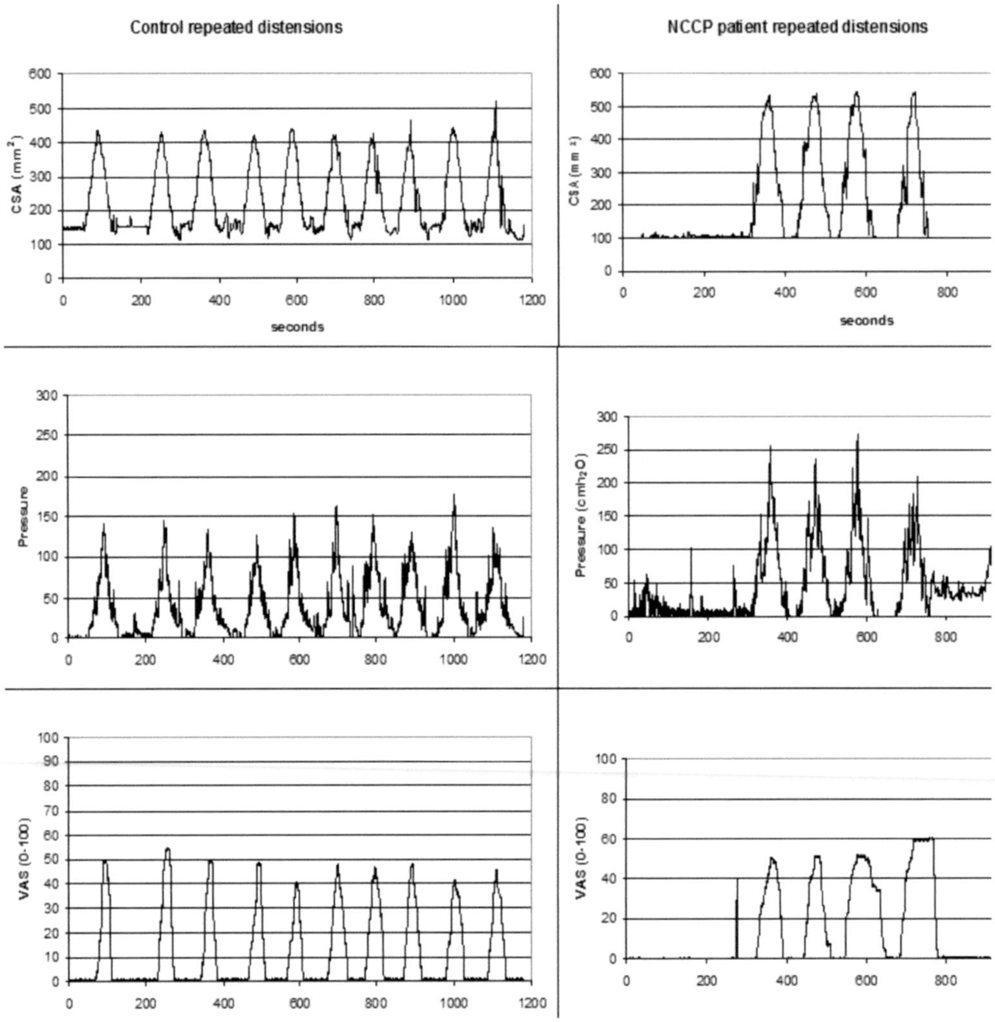

Figure 9: Data obtained during repeated distension of the esophagus in a healthy volunteer and a patient with non-cardiac chest pain. The distensions (pressure, cross-sectional area (CSA) and pain level (scale spanning from 0-100) were fairly reproducible in the healthy volunteer. The patient asked the examiner to stop after four distensions where especially the development in the VAS response differed from the healthy volunteer. Modified from Drewes *et al.* [60].

4.9. A STANDARDIZED METHOD FOR STUDYING TONE, SECONDARY PERISTALSIS AND THE MECHANISMS OF VISCERAL PAIN

This section describes a rather new method for obtaining the length-tension properties (the tension-strain diagram) of the gastrointestinal tract *in vivo*. This can be done by using balloon distension combined with impedance planimetry and proper distension protocols.

A bioengineer's approach to the analysis of gastrointestinal motor function requires the use of the available knowledge of the geometry and the material properties of the gastrointestinal tract, and the application of the basic laws of physics. In studying the effects of localized distension, a currently popular method to try to better define certain aspects of the system, we need both to use the stimulus accurately and to measure the response reliably. The new approach is based on controlled ramp bag distension along with the continuous determination of strain and tension in the organ wall under various conditions.

4.9.1. Probe Design and Distension Protocols

A four-electrode impedance measuring system (impedance planimeter) located inside a balloon on a 120-cm-long probe is used for measurements of CSA in the duodenum, antrum or esophagus (see chapter 3 for details on impedance planimetry). The attached balloon is 40 mm long and is made of 50-μm-thick non-conducting polyurethane. The balloon is connected through an infusion channel to a pump that can pump fluid in and out of the balloon at a variably controlled flow rate.

A pain questionnaire is given to all subjects to assess their visceral perceptions of the distension before the study starts. The balloon is positioned under fluoroscopic guidance in the third portion of the duodenum. Ramp-controlled distensions are then initiated at various volume rates, *e.g.* 25 ml per minute. The subjects are required to assess the intensity of their sensations continuously on a visual analog scale from zero to ten, where 0 is no sensation and 10 is unbearable pain. A visual analog scale rating of 5 is established as indicating the pain threshold. At a VAS rating of 5 or 7, the balloon is deflated at the same rate used for its inflation.

The tissue and the volunteer are first preconditioned. The distensions can be performed at different infusion speeds to test whether the receptors and the mechanical properties are strain-rate dependent. After a period of rest following one series of tests, the distensions can be repeated during the administration of the antimuscarinic drug butylscopolamine in sufficient doses to relax the smooth muscle. The total butylscopolamine dose to be used is guided by the degree of suppression of spontaneous contractions and by the development of classic anticholinergic side effects.

4.9.2. Computation of Active and Passive Tension

The circumferential wall tension (T) can be calculated according to the law of Laplace for cylindrical structures with the assumptions given in Chapter 2 or by other means. With imaging techniques it is potentially possible to compute average stresses rather than tensions. The total tension (T_{total}) during distension which is due both to active and passive tissue properties can be evaluated from the distension test without butylscopolamine administration. The passive tension ($T_{passive}$) resulting from passive components such as extracellular collagen is is assessed from the test with butylscopolamine or other muscle relaxing drugs (assuming that most activity can be removed). As a first approximation and assuming an additive relationship, the active tension (T_{active}) contributed by smooth muscle contraction can be computed using the equation

$$T_{total} = T_{active} + T_{passive} \tag{4.2}$$

The circumferential strain (ε) is the fractional change in radius computed as

$$\varepsilon = \frac{r - r_0}{r_0} \tag{4.3}$$

where r is the radius at a given distension and r_0 is the reference radius, ideally under unloaded mechanical conditions. The three tensions can be plotted as functions of strain to yield information about muscle function and tissue stiffness.

The volume, pressure, strain and tension are determined at the pain threshold (VAS = 5). The coefficient of variation (CV) can be computed as a statistical measure showing the relative variability of a trait to estimate which parameter the mechanoreceptors depend on at the pain threshold.

4.9.3. Active-Passive Tension-Strain Data obtained in the Human Duodenum of Young and Old Normal Subjects and Patients with Systemic Sclerosis

4.9.3.1. Normal Subjects

Studies have been conducted on the normal human duodenum [61].The length-tension diagrams were expressed in terms of tension-strain curves with distension rates of 25 ml min^{-1}. The total and passive tension increased as function of strain in an exponential manner. In contrast the active tension increased up to a maximum at a strain of 1.0. Active tension decreased at higher loads. The pain threshold appeared after the maximum on the tension strain curve was reached. From the data obtained in the study, it was clear that the sensation receptors respond both to the active tension (*i.e.* compression) and to circumferential stretch.

In some experiments, the volume is kept constant when VAS= 5 is reached during butylscopolamine infusion. In this case, it is observed that the perception intensity continues to increase after the infusion is stopped, *i.e.* while the volume and cross-sectional are not changing. It is seen, in fact, that the pressure diminishes because of stress relaxation. As a result, the passive tension also must decrease. Such data are, therefore, indicative of temporal summation.

The main conclusions that can be drawn at this time from these observations are: that the ramp-controlled balloon distension is applicable to intestinal studies in humans; that the passive elastic behavior is exponential; that, in the physiological range, the active tension curve influences the tissue behavior; and that the mechano-sensitive receptors in the duodenal wall react to circumferential wall strain rather than to volume, pressure or tension.

It was observed that the local active tension maximum always appeared before the gut wall was overstretched. The active component exhibited maximum tension development followed by a decline at higher degrees of stretch. This optimum tension is likely reached at the level of optimum overlap between the sliding filaments. The passive tension predominated when the pain threshold was reached. Hence, it seems the gastrointestinal tract wall can contribute its largest force to transport the bolus within the physiological range.

4.9.3.2. The Effect of Aging

Aging is considered to be a common reason for deterioration of organ function. Regarding the gastrointestinal tract, the following changes are sometimes said to occur as a result of aging:

- the total number of neurons in the myenteric plexus decreases, with an increase in the fibrous elements in the myenteric ganglia.

- the gastrointestinal muscle responds less well to excitatory agents, at least *in vitro.*

- neural injury in general may result from apoptosis, defects of mitochondrial metabolism, and inadequate levels or responses to neurotrophic substances.

- the morphology of collagen and the properties of the neuromuscular relationship change.

Changes like this could be expected to change the neural functions and biomechanical properties of the gastrointestinal tract.

The use of the new approach outlined above revealed that the pain threshold in the younger group was significantly higher for most mechanical parameters than those in the older subjects.

The unloaded size of the duodenum did not differ between younger and older subjects, but at higher loads it was found that the older group had lower CSA´s than the younger volunteers, indicating that the duodenal wall is stiffest in older people. The increase in stiffness was clearly confirmed in a comparison of the passive curves in the tension-strain graph; the passive tension curve was translated to the left for the older subjects when compared with the young subjects. Such a translation to the left in the coordinate system and a higher slope are consistent with a higher elastic modulus. In contrast, the pressure and tension of these two groups, both with and without administration of butylscopolamine, did not differ. The total and passive tension increased exponentially as function of strain or normalized volume in both groups. However, the active tension increased to a maximum at a strain of 0.6 in the older group and of approximately 1.0 in the younger group. This difference in strain was significant. The pain threshold appeared at a lower strain in the old group when compared to the young group.

The data demonstrate differences in the sensory and biomechanical properties of the duodenum between younger and older normal volunteers. The increased stiffness in older subjects may be associated with previous findings of a collagen accumulation in the intestine in old animal and human subjects since collagen has a high elastic modulus).

Other important findings relate to the local maximum in the active tension-strain curve. The tension recorded at the local maximum did not differ between the groups. This may be interpreted as that smooth muscle function is preserved in the older subjects since the muscle can generate a high active force. The maximum active tension, which is correlated with the smooth muscle contractile function, however, appeared at lower strain in the older subjects than in the younger. The mechanism for the shift in older individuals of the maximum towards a low strain is yet unknown However, a feasible explanation is resetting of the mechanosensitive receptors in the intestinal wall. Due to wall stiffening, the strain-sensitivity of the mechanoreceptors can likely reset as part of the structural and mechanical remodeling of the gastrointestinal tissue. It has yet to be determined whether this is a primary or secondary phenomenon. Since muscle function is preserved, the intestine does not appear to compensate for the lack of muscle contractile force. The data indicate the way in which his technique can explore these matters in biomechanical terms that have specific meanings with respect to specific biological functions.

4.9.3.3. Systemic Sclerosis

Systemic sclerosis is a rare disease characterized by an excessive deposition of collagen and other components of connective tissue in the skin and internal organs. The gastrointestinal tract is often involved with resultant structural changes and disturbances in motility. The change in proportion between smooth muscle and collagen in the intestinal wall should change its biomechanical properties. This remodeling of the gut wall is widely thought to explain the gastrointestinal dysfunction in systemic sclerosis patients.

Several papers have been published on the properties of esophagus and duodenum in patients with systemic sclerosis [62-67]. In similar experiments as those described above, it was found that total and passive tension both in the patients with systemic sclerosis and in controls increased exponentially as function of strain, and that the curves for the systemic sclerosis patients were shifted to the left. The excess extracellular matrix deposited in the intestinal wall may cause the increased stiffness since collagen has a high elastic modulus.

The active tension increased and reached a maximum at a strain of approximately 0.4 in the patients and of 0.6 in the age-matched healthy volunteers. Furthermore, the maximum active tension and the corresponding strain were higher in the healthy volunteers than in the patients with systemic sclerosis. The lower maximum tension in the systemic sclerosis patients indicates that the muscle is not capable of generating the same force as in volunteers. This is consistent with the known atrophy of the muscle layers and its replacement with collagen. The mechanism for the shift of the maximum towards a lower strain in the patients with systemic sclerosis is unknown from the present data, but resetting of the mechanosensitive receptors in the wall is a feasible explanation. Since the wall becomes stiffer, the strain-sensitivity of the mechanoreceptors may be reset as part of the remodeling of the tissue. It also seems feasible to propose that the intestine seeks to compensate for the lower maximum force generated by the muscle by initiating contractions at lower strains. The data indicate with more precision than was previously possible the changes in the biomechanics of the intestinal wall that occur in this disease.

Another major finding is that the systemic sclerosis patients had higher perception score than the normal subjects when they underwent the same level of mechanical stimulation. This suggests that the pain receptor located in the duodenal wall in patients with systemic sclerosis is hypersensitive, perhaps through receptor resetting.

4.9.3.4. Conclusions and Perspectives

It is possible to study the relation between the biomechanical behavior of the human small intestine and the sensations that arise from its distension. The data indicate the following:

- The smooth muscle length-tension diagram known from studies *in vitro* can be reproduced from studies of the human intestine *in vivo*.
- The mechanoreceptors located in the gastrointestinal wall depend on wall circumferential strain rather than intraluminal volume and pressure and wall tension; also, the high threshold receptors are non-adapting.
- Aging results in stiffening of the duodenal wall and in resetting of the receptors in the gut. These changes accompany hypersensitivity to distension in aging.

- The duodenum of patients with systemic sclerosis is stiffer and shows less motor activity than normal subjects. The intestinal wall in systemic sclerosis patients is hypersensitive.

Pain is a multi-dimensional, highly individual perception, with cognitive and emotional aspects, that is difficult to quantify and to validate. Experimental models in humans may improve our understanding of visceral pain mechanisms. Such models have been hard to develop because of the inaccessibility of the viscera.

Mechanical stimulation by distension of the gut with a balloon seems to mimic, in part, the symptoms of mechanical obstruction of the gut. Hence, the use of such models might reveal something about the pain system of the gut. The mechanical stimulus, however, needs to be well defined and reproducible, as is the case in this new technique. This new method demonstrates the possibilities it offers for revealing specific aspects or characteristics of a mechanical system, the gastrointestinal tract, which, heretofore, has suffered from neglect by the only discipline that can describe it, mechanics.

Part of this chapter has been previously published in Complex Anorectal Disorders, 2005, pp. 72-104.

REFERENCES

[1] Hill AV. First and last experiments in muscle mechanics. Cambridge University Press 1970.

[2] Fung YC. Biomechanics: Mechanical properties of living tissues. New York: Springer-Verlag 1993.

[3] Macagno EO, Christensen J. Fluid mechanics of gastrointestinal flow. In: Physiology of the gastrointestinal tract. LR Johnson *et al*, Eds. New York, Raven Press 1981.

[4] Pal A, Brasseur JG. The mechanical advantage of local longitudinal shortening on peristaltic transport. J Biomech Eng 2002; 124: 94-100

[5] Fackler K, Klein L, Hiltner AJ. Polarizing light microscopy of intestine and its relationship to mechanical behavior. J Microsc 1981; 124: 305-311.

[6] Orberg J, Baer E, Hiltner A. Organization of collagen fibers in the intestine. Conn Tiss Res 1983; 11: 285-297.

[7] Fung YC. Biomechanics: Motion, Flow, Stress, and Growth. New York; Springer-Verlag 1990.

[8] Fung YC, Liu SQ. Changes of residual strains in arteries due to hypertrophy caused by aortic constriction. Circulation Research 1989; 65: 1340-1349.

[9] Gregersen H, Kassab GS. Biomechanics of the gastrointestinal tract. Neurogastroenterol Motility 1996; 8: 277-297.

[10] Gregersen H. Biomechanics of the Gastrointestinal Tract. Springer Verlag. London. 2002.

[11] Gregersen H, Kassab G, Pallencaoe E, Lee C, Chien S, Skalak R, Fung YC. Morphometry and strain distribution in guinea pig duodenum with reference to the zero-stress state. Am J Physiol 1997; 273: G865-G874.

[12] Gregersen H, Kassab GS, Fung YC. The zero-stress state of the gastrointestinal tract: biomechanical and functional implications. Digestive Diseases and Science 2000; 45: 2271-2281.

[13] Gregersen H, Lee C, Chien S, Skalak R, Fung YC. Strain distribution in the layered wall of the esophagus. J Biomed Eng 1999; 121: 442-448.

[14] Gregersen H. Residual strain in the gastrointestinal tract: A new concept. Neurogastroenterol Motility 2000; 12: 411-414.

[15] Rodriguez EK, Hoger A, McCulloch AD. Stress-dependent finite growth in soft elastic tissues. J Biomech 1994; 27: 455-467.

[16] Lu X, Zhao J, Gregersen H. Small intestinal morphometric and biomechanical changes during physiological growth in rats. J Biomech 2005; 38: 417-26.

[17] Gregersen H, Lu X, Zhao J. Physiological growth is associated with esophageal morphometric and biomechanical changes in rats. Neurogastroenterol Motil 2004; 16: 403-412.

[18] Dou Y, Gregersen S, Zhao J, Zhuang F, Gregersen H. Morphometric and biomechanical intestinal remodeling induced by fasting in rats. Dig Dis Sci 2002; 47:1158-1168.

[19] Dou Y, Gregersen S, Zhao J, Zhuang F, Gregersen H. Effect of re-feeding after starvation on biomechanical properties in rat small intestine. Med Eng Phys 2001; 23: 557-566.

[20] Gregersen H[1], Weis SM, McCulloch AD. Oesophageal morphometry and residual strain in a mouse model of osteogenesis imperfecta. Neurogastroenterol Motil 2001; 13: 457-464.

[21] Zhao J, Chen P, Gregersen H. Stress-strain analysis of jejunal contractility in response to flow and ramp distension in type 2 diabetic GK rats: effect of carbachol stimulation. J Biomech 2013; 46: 2469-2476.

[22] Zhao J, Chen P, Gregersen H. Morpho-mechanical intestinal remodeling in type 2 diabetic GK rats--is it related to advanced glycation end product formation. J Biomech 2013; 46: 1128-1134.

[23] Liu GF, Zhao JB, Zhen Z, Sha H, Chen PM, Li M, Zhang JC, Yuan MZ, Gao W, Gregersen H, Tong XL. Effect of tangweian jianji on upper gastrointestinal remodeling in streptozotocin-induced diabetic rats. World J Gastroenterol 2012; 18: 4875-4884.

[24] Zhao J, Yang J, Vinter-Jensen L, Zhuang F, Gregersen H. Biomechanical properties of esophagus during systemic treatment with epidermal growth factor in rats. Ann Biomed Eng 2003; 31: 700-709.

[25] Yang J, Zhao J, Zeng Y, Vinter-Jensen L, Gregersen H. Morphological properties of zero-stress state in rat large intestine during systemic EGF treatment. Dig Dis Sci 2003; 48: 442-8.

[26] Liao D, Yang J, Zhao J, Zeng Y, Vinter-Jensen L, Gregersen H.The effect of epidermal growth factor on the incremental Young's moduli in the rat small intestine. Med Eng Phys 2003; 25: 413-418.

[27] Zhao J, Yang J, Vinter-Jensen L, Zhuang F, Gregersen H. The morphometry and biomechanical properties of the rat small intestine after systemic treatment with epidermal growth factor. Biorheology 2002; 39: 719-733.

[28] Vinter-Jensen L, Duch BU, Petersen JA, Ryslev A, Gregersen H. Systemic treatment with epidermal growth factor in the rat. Biomechanical properties of the growing small intestine. Regul Pept 1996; 61: 135-142

[29] Lu C, Schulze-Delrieu K, Shirazi S, Cram M, Raab J. Dynamic imaging of obstructed opossum esophagus. From altered load to altered contractility. Dig Dis Sci 1994; 39: 1377-1388.

[30] Tung HN, Shirazi S, Schulze-Delrieu K, Brown K. Morphological changes of myenteric neurons in the partially obstructed opossum esophagus. J Submicrosc Cytol Pathol 1993; 25: 357-363.

[31] Tung HN, Schulze-Delrieu K, Shirazi S. Infiltration of hypertrophic esophageal smooth muscle by mast cells and basophils. J Submicrosc Cytol Pathol 1993; 25: 93-102.

[32] Zhao J, Liao D, Yang J, Gregersen H. Phasic and tonic smooth muscle function of the partially obstructed guinea pig intestine. J Biomed Biotechnol 2011; 48: 97-120.

[33] Zhao J, Liao D, Yang J, Gregersen H. Stress and strain analysis of contractions during ramp distension in partially obstructed guinea pig jejunal segments. J Biomech 2011; 44: 2077-2082.

[34] Liao D, Zhao J, Gregersen H. 3d Mechanical properties of the partially obstructed guinea pig small intestine. J Biomech 2010; 43: 2079-2086.

[35] Zhao J, Liao D, Yang J, Gregersen H. Biomechanical remodelling of obstructed guinea pig jejunum. J Biomech 2010; 43: 1322-1329.

[36] Storkholm JH, Zhao J, Villadsen GE, Gregersen H. Spontaneous and bolus-induced motility in the chronically obstructed guinea-pig small intestine *in vitro*. Dig Dis Sci 2008; 53: 413-20.

[37] Storkholm JH, Zhao J, Villadsen GE, Hager H, Jensen SL, Gregersen H. Biomechanical remodeling of the chronically obstructed Guinea pig small intestine. Dig Dis Sci 2007; 52: 336-346.

[38] Gabella G. Structural apparatus for force transmission in smooth muscles. Physiological Reviews 1984; 64: 455-477.

[39] Gabella G. Structure of muscles and nerves in the gastrointestinal tract. In: Physiology of the Gastrointestinal Tract. Johnson LR, Christensen J, Jackson MJ, Jacobson ED, Walsh JH, Eds. New York, Raven Press 1987; pp. 335-382.

[40] Duch BU, Andersen HL, Smith J, Kassab GS, Gregersen H. Structural and mechanical remodelling of the common bile duct after obstruction. Neurogastroenterol Motil 2002; 14: 111-122.

[41] Duch BU, Andersen H, Gregersen H. Morphometric and biomechanical remodelling following reopening of the obstructed bile duct. Physiol Meas 2003; 24: N23-34.

[42] Senn N. An Experimental Contribution to Intestinal Surgery, with Special Reference to the Treatment of Intestinal Obstruction (Concluded). Ann Surg 1888; 7: 421-430.

[43] Dou Y, Lu X, Zhao J, Gregersen H. Morphometric and biomechanical remodelling in the intestine after small bowel resection in the rat. Neurogastroenterol Motil 2004; 14: 43-53.

[44] Li M, Brasseur JG, Kern MK, *et al.* Viscosity measurements of barium sulfate mixtures for use in motility studies of the pharynx and esophagus. Dysphagia 1992; 7: 17-30.

[45] Brasseur JG. Mechanical studies of the esophageal function. Dysphagia 1993; 8: 384-386.

[46] Christensen J. The Motility of the Colon. In: Johnson LR, Alpers DH, Christensen J, Jacobson ED, Walsh JH, Eds. Physiology of the Gastrointestinal Tract. 3rd edition, New York, Raven Press1994; pp. 991-1024.

[47] Stavitsky D, Macagno EO, Christensen J. Finite-element analysis of flow induced by contractions like those of the intestine. J Biomech 1981; 14: 183-193.

[48] Miftakhov RN, Abdusheva GR, Christensen J. Numerical Simulation of Motility Patterns of the Small Bowel. Part I-Formulation of a Mathematical Model. J Theoretical Biology 1999; 197: 89-112.

[49] Miftakhov RN, Wingate DL. Numerical Simulation of the Peristaltic Reflex of the Small Bowel. J Biorheologyn 1994; 31: 309-325.

[50] Trendelenburg P. Physiological and pharmacological investigations of small intestinal peristalsis. Translation of the article "Physiologische und pharmakologische Versuche über die

Dünndarmperistaltik", Arch Exp Pathol Pharmakol 1917; 81:55-129. Naunyn Schmiedebergs Arch Pharmacol 2006; 373: 101-33.

[51] Gregersen H, Christensen J. Gastrointestinal Tone. Neurogastroenterol Motility 2000; 12: 501-508.

[52] Mandrek K, Golenhofen K. Tonic duodenal contractions - a process for regulation of duodenal transit. In: Frontiers in smooth muscle research. Alan R. Liss, Inc. 1990; pp.459-462.

[53] Szymanski PT, Chacko TK, Rovner AS, Goyal RK. Differences in contractile protein content and isoforms in phasic and tonic smooth muscle. Am J Physiol 1998; 275: C684-C692.

[54] Christensen J, Torres EI. Three layers of the opossum stomach: responses to nerve stimulation. Gastroenterology 1975; 69: 641-648.

[55] Gregersen H, Orvar K, Christensen J. Biomechanical wall properties and tone during phase I and phase II of the MMC. Am J Physiol 1992; 263: G795-G801.

[56] Mayrand S, Tremblay L, Diamant N. *In vivo* measurement of feline esophageal tone. Am J Physiol 1994; 267: G914-21.

[57] Mayrand S, Diamant NE. Measurement of human esophageal tone *in vivo*. Gastroenterology 1993; 105: 1411-1420.

[58] Paton WD, Vane JR. Analysis of the responses of the isolated stomach to electrical stimulation and to drugs. J Physiol 1963; 165: 10-46

[59] Ødegaard S, Gilja OH, Gregersen H. Basic and New aspects of Gastrointestinal Ultrasonography. Singapore: World Scientific Publishers 2005.

[60] Drewes AM, Pedersen J, Reddy H, Rasmussen K, Funch-Jensen P, Arendt-Nielsen L, Gregersen H. Central sensitization in patients with non-cardiac chest pain: A clinical experimental pain study. World J Gastroenterol 2006; 41; 640-649.

[61] Gao C, Arendt-Nielsen L, Liu W, Petersen P, Drewes AM, Gregersen H. Sensory and biomechanical responses to ramp-controlled distension of the human duodenum. Am J Physiol Gastrointest Liver Physiol 2003; 284: G461-71

[62] Gregersen H, Villadsen GE, Liao D. Mechanical characteristics of distension-evoked peristaltic contractions in the esophagus ofsystemic sclerosis patients. Dig Dis Sci 2011; 56: 3559-3568.

[63] Gao F, Liao D, Drewes AM, Gregersen H. Modelling the elastin, collagen and smooth muscle contribution to the duodenal mechanical behaviour in patients with systemic sclerosis. Neurogastroenterol Motil 2009; 21: 914-e68.

[64] Gregersen H, Liao D, Pedersen J, Drewes AM. A new method for evaluation of intestinal muscle contraction properties: studies in normal subjects and in patients with systemic sclerosis. Neurogastroenterol Motil 2007; 19: 11-19.

[65] Pedersen J, Gao C, Egekvist H, Bjerring P, Arendt-Nielsen L, Gregersen H, Drewes AM. Pain and biomechanical responses to distention of the duodenum in patients with systemic sclerosis. Gastroenterology 2003; 124: 1230-1239.

[66] Villadsen GE, Storkholm J, Zachariae H, Hendel L, Bendtsen F, Gregersen H. Oesophageal pressure-cross-sectional area distributions and secondary peristalsis in relation to subclassification of systemic sclerosis. Neurogastroenterol Motil 2001; 13: 199-210.

[67] Villadsen GE, Storkholm JH, Hendel L, Vilstrup H, Gregersen H. Impedance planimetric characterization of esophagus in systemic sclerosis patients with severe involvement of esophagus. Dig Dis Sci 1997; 42: 2317-2326.

CHAPTER 5

The Mechanical System: Motor Patterns in Organs

Abstract: The mechanical systems of the gut must move nutrients in whatever complex ways may be necessary in each situation for digestive and absorptive processes to be complete. The mechanical processes vary from one species to another but they differ mainly in quantitative rather than qualitative terms. This chapter deals with the movements of the gastrointestinal musculature throughout the tract. Most of these patterns of motion are inferred rather that observed directly, for the available methods rarely permit the direct and detailed observation of the muscular behavior *in vivo*.

Keywords: Contractility, esophagus, flow, large intestine, motility pattern, peristalsis, relaxation, small intestine, stomach.

5.1. INTRODUCTION

The nutritional needs of the organism require that the gastrointestinal tract must be able to convert whatever food is available to the animal into the simple molecules that can be used by the tissues of the body. In order to serve this function, the gastrointestinal tract evolved in various ways to accommodate the many different kinds of foodstuffs available to different classes of animals.

Thus, the alimentary canal varies enormously in its configuration among the different kinds of animals. The gut in aquatic animals differs structurally from that in terrestrial animals. The gastrointestinal tract of herbivorous animals differs greatly from that of carnivorous animals. Even within the herbivores, major anatomic differences, especially notable in the stomach, distinguish the ruminants from the other sorts of herbivores. Birds have distinctive nutritional machinery that also varies with their diets. The human gastrointestinal tract (Fig. **1**) is the subject of this chapter.

The mechanical systems of the gut must move nutrients in whatever complex ways may be necessary in each situation for digestive and absorptive processes to be complete. Fundamental mechanisms operate in all animals, however, despite the major structural differences. The mechanical (and biochemical) processes vary from one species to another but they differ mainly in quantitative rather than qualitative terms.

Hans Gregersen and James Christensen

In all species, the motions of the walls must

- accomplish net antegrade flow
- reduce ingested materials to a suitable homogeneous fluid
- mix the luminal fluids
- move fluid across the luminal surface where secretion and nutrient absorption occurs, and
- remove undigested residue

These goals require that the motor mechanisms move the ingesta appropriately both into and out of the separate organs that are dedicated to the special functions involved in alimentation. Since the organs act in concert rather than in independence, regulatory and coordinating mechanisms are critical.

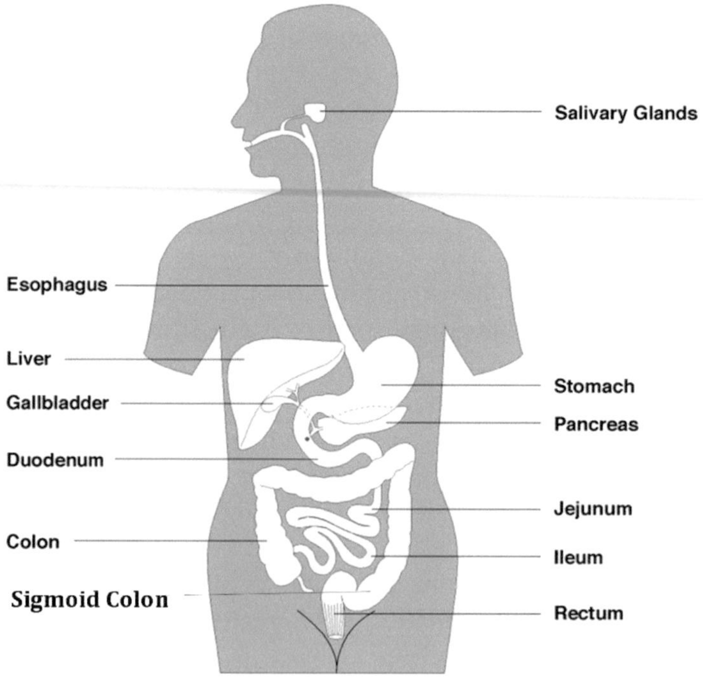

Figure 1: A scheme showing the viscera of the gastrointestinal tract in man and indicating their relative sizes and positions.

Much gastrointestinal disease represents, in part, the abnormal movement of the contents from one region into another. Even in gallstone disease, a clinical disorder that seems, on the face of it, not to involve motor mechanisms, the stones arise in part from the abnormal flow of bile and, once formed, they also affect that flow.

So intimately is motility tied to the secretory and absorptive functions of the gut that these three general operations cannot be seriously considered separately, except in highly reductionist thinking. Medical science, however, commonly ignores motor mechanisms in considering gastrointestinal disorders. This happens in large part, probably, because motor mechanisms are so poorly comprehended by medical science.

It is a common concept among naive persons that gastrointestinal motility consists basically of intermittent periods in which short annular constrictions, circumferential narrowings of a cylindrical soft-shelled conduit, move at a uniform velocity and occur at a uniform frequency. Also, in the common view, short and stationary annular constrictions (sphincters), regulated independently, lie at the conjunctions of adjacent organs both to regulate antegrade flow and to prevent retrograde flow. Besides being simplistic and wrong, this concept gives no account of the operations of the muscle layers other than the circular layer.

Such a naive and erroneous scheme arose from the limited research in this subject area in the 19th century, and it became entrenched. It stems also from the persistent inclination to view the alimentary canal in analogy to familiar hydraulic systems that involve pumps, pipes and valves. This is understandable because the human mind works naturally by seeking analogies. However, the complex mechanisms and flows that actually occur in the gastrointestinal tract defy such easy comparisons to familiar devices or manufactured systems for the management of fluids. A more realistic understanding is necessary if our management of the disorders of the system is to be improved.

A most important overview about the mechanical system is the fact that three muscle layers exist in all organs (except for the pharynx). The variety of deformations of the wall that can be produced by the simultaneous operation of the three muscle layers defies description in the absence of knowledge about their interactions and patterns of behavior. Still, common sense allows one to make some important generalizations:

- The circular muscle layer, because its contraction occludes the lumen, must affect especially the net translocation of luminal contents along the axis of the conduit and so it could affect both the propulsive and the resistive forces in axial flow.

- The arrangement of the mucosal muscle indicates that it must move the mobile mucosa in the plane of the inner surface of the conduit, enhancing the circulation of luminal contents over the surface of the mucosa.

- The longitudinal muscle layer must tend to shorten segments of the gut when it contracts, and it must stiffen the wall of the conduit; At any single point (at least in the esophagus) this layer contracts before the circular muscle layer does and its contraction outlasts that of the circular layer so that it stiffens and thickens the wall before the peristaltic contraction occurs and that action may enhance the force of peristalsis.

- The three muscle layers might sometimes operate independently, but it seems most likely that they usually work together in each organ to accomplish a purpose that requires their conjoined efforts through the offices of an integrating system, the intrinsic innervation of the gut.

  Since the major purpose of each organ is a little different, the motions of the wall must vary from one organ to another. This indicates the existence of variation among organs in the behavior of the muscle. This fact implies, also, the existence of differences in the nature of the regulating system of nerves from one organ to another.

This chapter deals with the movements of the gastrointestinal musculature throughout the tract. Most of these patterns of motion are inferred rather that observed directly, for the available methods now rarely permit the direct and detailed observation of the muscular behavior *in vivo*. The evidence that leads to these conclusions comes from a diverse array of techniques and disciplines but the descriptions given here generally explain all the evidence, whatever its nature. In most cases, the physical scientist would seek a more quantitative description than that provided here. In some such instances, the available methods cannot give more quantitation, but they allow approximations or reasonable assumptions to be made. In other cases the need for quantification simply has not been sufficiently recognized. The reader is referred to general textbooks for further reading of background literature on the general motor patterns. In addition references [1-8] are informative.

5.2. PHARYNX AND PHARYNGOESOPHAGEAL SPHINCTER

5.2.1. The Organ "at Rest"

5.2.1.1. The Pharyngeal Constrictors

The pharynx serves two mechanical functions. In swallowing, it carries food from the mouth to the esophagus through complex motions induced by the contractions of the muscle of its walls. At rest, it serves for the passage of air to and from the lungs in respiration. Thus, at rest, it need not move but must be open to let the air pass.

The three layers of pharyngeal muscle in the resting state maintain a fairly stable partial contraction. This condition of stable shortening, muscle tone, is low enough to allow the pharynx to remain open as a part of the airway, but great enough to reduce the size of the organ so that no significant pooling of salivary secretions occurs there.

As in all somatic muscles (where tone is an almost universal property), the maintained contracted state of the three overlapping pharyngeal constrictors represents a constant low level of discharge of the excitatory motor nerves to the muscle, the somatic motor fibers of the ninth cranial (glossopharynbgeal) nerves. The constancy of the muscle tone reflects the existence of a regulatory neural mechanism that maintains the equilibrium of the neural excitation. The firing of the excitatory nerves must originate in the cell bodies of those motor nerves, which are located in the motor nuclei of the brainstem.

There are two such ninth cranial nerves, right and left, each innervating the corresponding half of the pharyngeal musculature. The pharynx is symmetrical at rest as well as in movement. This symmetry in pharyngeal form and movement means that the regulatory mechanisms in the two sides must be exactly coordinated in their operation, probably through connections from the nuclei of the ninth cranial nerve on one side of the brainstem to those on the other.

The stability of pharyngeal muscle tone must reflect a corresponding stability in the rate of the neural discharge in the motor fibers of the ninth nerve. The rate at which the nerves fire seems most likely to depend upon a feedback mechanism that monitors the force being exerted by the contraction of the muscle cells and uses that information to control the firing rate of the excitatory nerves. The monitors are almost certainly the special sensory structures located in this musculature, the muscle spindles, which serve as mechanoreceptors. These spindles are the terminals of sensory nerve fibers that lie within of the ninth cranial nerves. They must transmit their information to centers within the brainstem that establish the limits of the range of tone allowed at rest. That is, the rate of tonic discharge of the mechanoreceptors probably determines the rate of tonic discharge of the motor fibers. This functional analysis rests almost entirely upon conjecture from anatomical evidence.

5.2.1.2. The Pharyngoesophageal Sphincter

As a part of the inferior constrictor of the pharynx, this sphincter must possess the same regulatory mechanisms that the three pharyngeal constrictors do. Its function, however, differs a little.

At rest, it maintains a contraction that exerts just enough force at the pharyngoesophageal junction to occlude the lumen. In this way, the sphincter separates the pharyngeal lumen from the esophageal lumen at rest. This closure prevents the entry of air into the esophagus during respiration and keeps esophageal content from entering the respiratory tract.

The pharyngoesophageal sphincter is so short that its length during tonic contraction at rest approximates the shortest distance between its origin and insertion, the two ends of the cricoid cartilage. This single anatomic fact explains why this sphincter fully occludes the lumen at rest while the adjacent pharyngeal constrictors do not. In contracting, the sphincter can thus close the passage even when the force of that contraction is only just enough to keep the muscle from flaccidity. It occludes by lateral compression of the lumen to produce a slit. Some evidence indicates that a mechanism exists for the regulation of the force of this tonic contraction: the force at rest can be made to change through the activation of sensory nerves in the rostral part of the esophagus.

5.2.1.3. The Parapharyngeal Muscles (The Strap Muscles of the Neck)

A set of complexly named muscles, collectively called the parapharyngeal muscles, controls the position of the pharynx within the neck. These muscles attach the pharyngoesophageal conduit to the base of the skull through their origin, directly and indirectly, on the skull and their insertion on the bony structures in the pharyngoesophageal conduit, the hyoid bone and the laryngeal cartilage.

They exhibit tone at rest, the stable state of partial contraction found in somatic muscle generally. This tone keeps the position of the pharyngoesophageal junction constant and maintains a reasonably constant angle between the lumen of the pharynx and that of the esophagus. These factors discourage the passage of pharyngeal content into the esophagus, consistent with the normal flow of air in breathing. The mechanism for the stability of the tone in the strap muscles seems to be the same as that which operates in the pharyngeal constrictors (see above).

5.2.2. The Organ in Action

The initiation of a swallow involves the familiar volitional movements of the jaw, tongue, and soft palate. These movements activate mechanoreceptors in those structures to trigger the discharge of the neurons of the swallowing center, a physically unidentified organizational unit in the brainstem. This center coordinates the discharge of the brainstem motor nuclei to accomplish the subsequent involuntary movements of the pharynx and esophagus in swallowing.

5.2.2.1. The Pharyngeal Constrictors

The initial response of the pharyngeal constrictors to a swallow is a very brief loss of the stable tone that they manifest at rest. This relaxation is so brief as to have no appreciable effect on the gross configuration of the organ. This brief and inapparent inhibition in stable discharge of the motor innervation, however, is followed by a powerful discharge of the same nerves, producing a strong contraction. The contraction seems to represent a rebound of the nerves to the antecedent inhibition.

The contraction begins first in the superior constrictor, passing rapidly to the others in craniocaudal sequence and moving throughout the whole organ. It occludes the pharyngeal lumen completely. The progressive nature of the contraction could have either of two explanations:

- The activation could begin at essentially the same moment throughout each muscle mass, each of the three constrictors, but the activation of three muscles could be successively delayed with a phase lag in the rostrocaudal direction. That is, each constrictor could contract unitarily a little later than its rostral companion does.

- The activation could move as a front through each constrictor with a successive delay from one point to the next within each muscle mass.

The fact that the motor units of pharyngeal muscle are small, as small as those of the finest somatic muscles, such as the extraocular muscles, supports the latter idea. A motor unit is a single somatic motor nerve fiber together with the number of striated muscle cells innervated by that fiber. It represents the adjacent muscle cells that must contract simultaneously when that motor neuron discharges. The number of muscle cells regulated by a single motor neuron is fixed. The number of muscle cells in a motor unit varies among different somatic muscles. The motor unit in this musculature is estimated to be a matter of ten cells or so, the size of motor units in the finest somatic muscles such as the extra ocular muscles.

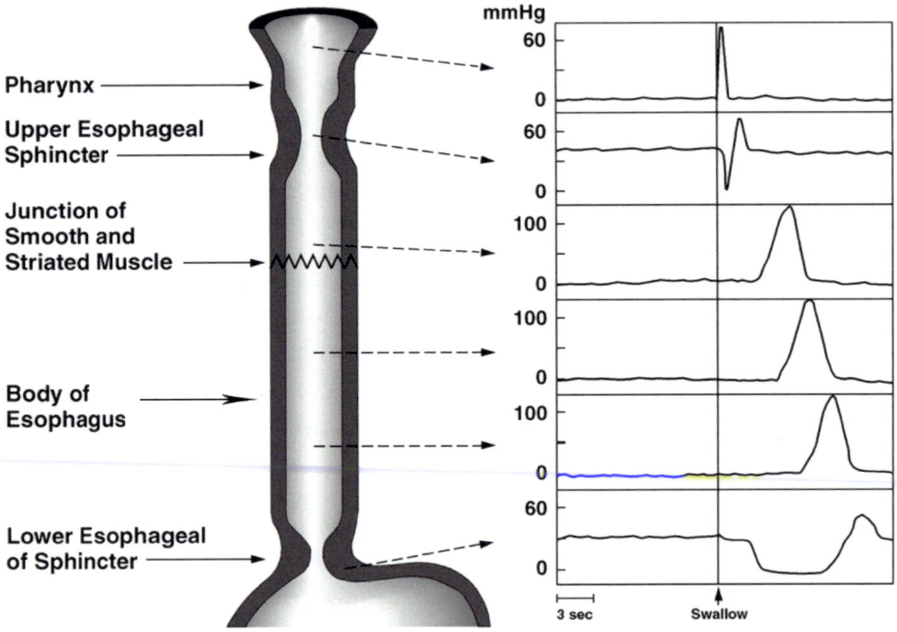

Figure 2: A drawing to show the sequence of contractions that occur in the pharynx and esophagus after a swallow. The organs are shown at the left while the column of tracings at the right represent the intraluminal pressure as measured at six points at the levels indicated by the dashed lines with an arrowhead. The sketch shows that pharyngeal contraction is followed successively by relaxation of the pharyngoesophageal sphincter and a peristaltic contraction that moves uniformly throughout the esophagus. The gastroesophageal sphincter relaxes early in the process and contracts as the peristaltic contraction reaches it. Nowadays contraction sequences in the esophagus is often shown as color contour plots using high resolution manometry.

In any case, the rostrocaudal movement of the contraction is determined in the swallowing center in the brainstem, not peripherally. It is the result of a triggered and stereotyped program, apparently unaffected by sensory inputs other than those that initiate it. That is, once triggered, the pattern of neuronal discharge seems to be invariant. The same program regulates the operation of the pharyngo-esophageal sphincter (Fig. **2**).

5.2.2.2. The Pharyngoesophageal Sphincter

The neurogenic inhibition that precedes the swallowing-induced contraction of the striated muscle in the pharynx has a crucial role in the function of the pharyngoesophageal sphincter, whereas it has no obvious effect on the mechanics of the main body of the pharynx.

The initiation of a swallow makes the muscle of this sphincter relax so that it offers no hindrance to the opening of the lumen by a bolus pressed into it by the pharyngeal muscle contraction. Because the sphincter is actually a part of the inferior constrictor, it is not surprising that the sphincter contracts vigorously at the end of its relaxation in a swallow. The sphincter actually goes through the same sequence of events as the pharyngeal constrictors, a relaxation followed by a contraction. The difference between the two structures is that the major function of the pharyngeal constrictors is the contractile component of the event whereas the relaxing component is the principal feature in the pharyngoesophageal sphincter. The contraction in the sphincter, after it has relaxed briefly, exerts a large force after which the muscle quickly returns to the lower but stable (tonic) force that characterizes the resting state.

The tone of this sphincter at rest accomplishes the critical purpose of maintaining the closure of the lumen into the esophagus, thus helping to keep the airway separated from the gastrointestinal tract. This barrier function, however, is shared with a number of other mechanisms so that the destruction of the sphincter alone does not lead to the entry of foodstuffs into the airway. The other mechanisms that operate in a swallow to keep food out of the airway include pharyngeal shortening and reorientation in the neck, and the symmetry of pharyngeal peristalsis. In most diseases that destroy the sphincter, however, these other factors are also disturbed so that abnormal diversion of food into the airway can occur.

5.2.2.3. The Parapharyngeal Muscles (The Strap Muscles of the Neck)

The tone in the parapharyngeal muscles at rest holds the pharynx, esophagus, and the larynx at such a position in the midline of the neck that the angle of insertion of the pharynx into the esophagus discourages the passage of pharyngeal content into that opening. When the parapharyngeal muscles are activated after the initiation of a swallow, they first relax very briefly and then they contract strongly, like the rest of the somatic musculature of this system. This contraction moves the organs to align the axis of the esophageal lumen more closely with that of the pharynx, facilitating passage from the one to the other. This alignment takes place at the same time that the three pharyngeal constrictors contract and the pharyngoesophageal sphincter relaxes.

5.2.3. The Program for Pharyngeal Function

The entire program for these events lies in the brainstem. The structures that carry out the program are identifiable as the recognized anatomic structures (nuclei and tracts) long ago named by neuroanatomists. The ways in which they work within themselves and within their functional interconnections, however, remains to be clarified. So many different kinds of structures participate in process of swallowing that a "swallowing center", an organizing core has been postulated, but the details of its physical nature remain as obscure as those of its functional character. Only the final results of the output of the center can be readily observed and so the nature of its operations must be inferred from those outputs.

The pharyngeal motor events are triggered wholly through the ninth cranial (glossopharyngeal) nerves, with unilateral representation in both the right and left neural centers in the organ. That is, the nerve fibers from the each side pass only to the musculature of that side. There appears to be essentially no crossover of nerve fibers from one side to the other within the pharyngeal wall. Thus, the swallowing center must trigger the discharge of the nuclei of both sides essentially simultaneously, but firing only when the need for certain sensory inputs to the swallowing center have been satisfied. These preconditions seem to include inputs from sensory nerves that deliver information from mechanoreceptors in the musculature of the face, tongue, and jaws.

The nuclei of the ninth cranial nerve also serve the striated muscle for a short distance into the upper esophagus where there is an overlap with the distribution of the motor nerves emanating from the tenth cranial nerves (the vagus nerves). The discharge of the tenth cranial nerve nuclei comes well after that of the ninth cranial nerve nuclei so that the consequence of their coordinated discharge, the mechanical operation of the pharynx and esophagus, appears as a smooth and uniform process (Fig. **2**).

The progression of the contraction front through the striated muscle of the pharynx must represent the serial discharge of motor units in a craniocaudal sequence. No other explanation for the progression is possible because of the fact that the innervation of somatic muscle throughout the body follows the pattern of a motor unit organization.

5.2.4. Pharyngeal Flow

At the initiation of a swallow, which is voluntary, the tongue pushes a bolus into the upper end of the oropharynx. The elevation of the soft palate (produced by the muscle contraction) separates the nasopharynx from the oropharynx so that contraction of the pharyngeal constrictors can displace this bolus only toward the esophagus.

The bolus flows rapidly. If it consists of a thin liquid, it may flow so fast under the hydrostatic force that it reaches the pharyngoesophageal sphincter almost as soon as the pharyngeal contraction has begun. Even then, it arrives after the sphincter has relaxed because the relaxation in this complex of muscles always precedes the contraction. In that case, the bolus shoots as a jet into the esophageal opening. If the liquid bolus arrives too soon, before the sphincter has fully relaxed or before the strap muscles have fully realigned the viscera, it enters the larynx, an abnormal event called aspiration or laryngeal penetration.

The duration of the relaxation-contraction sequence in the pharyngeal muscles assures that solid masses, which move through the organ largely under the influence of the pharyngeal contraction, also reach the sphincter while it is still relaxed. Thus, the bolus normally passes through the sphincter with no delay and completes its passage before the sphincter regains its tonic closure. However, a small fraction of the bolus may normally linger in the pharynx, especially when it contains viscous liquids. Such fluids commonly remain in small pockets that result from the way the organ is constructed, the pyriform sinuses or valleculae. A prompt second swallow, often produced virtually as a reflex event, normally empties these pockets immediately.

5.3. ESOPHAGUS AND ESOPHAGOGATRIC SPHINCTER

5.3.1. The Organ "at Rest"

5.3.1.1. The Esophageal Body

Between swallows, the esophagus remains stable. The flaccid wall of the esophageal body (the long segment between the pharyngoesophageal and esophagogastric sphincters) exhibits only passive movements, a result of the motions of cardiac events and the motions of the chest in breathing. The midline position of the esophagus in the thorax minimizes the displacements provoked by such external forces.

Both the striated muscle of the upper third of the organ and the visceral muscle of the rest of the organ (except for the esophagogastric sphincter) exhibit a low degree of tone. In sharp contrast, the latter sphincter, the thickened zone in the circular muscle layer just above the junction to the stomach, exhibits enough tone to occlude the lumen at this level. At rest, the closed pharyngoesophageal sphincter and the esophagogastric sphincter together respectively separate the lumen of the flaccid esophageal body from the atmosphere and from the stomach. Thus, the fluctuating pressure in the empty esophageal lumen remains subatmospheric, reflecting intrathoracic pressure.

Normally, the lumen of the esophageal body at rest contains nothing but a little air and a very small quantity of saliva, enough to coat the luminal surface. A stable tension, called residual stress, exists in the wall that is capable of buckling the mucosa. This intramural tension, possibly arising from passive properties of that layer, is sufficient to throw the mucosa into longitudinal folds that come together at the center of the organ, especially in the most caudal few centimeters. They may serve to weakly oppose gastroesophageal reflux rostral to the esophagogastric sphincter.

5.3.1.2. The Esophagogastric Sphincter

This sphincter is the short segment of the organ just above the stomach in which the circular muscle layer appears to be slightly thicker than it is elsewhere in the organ. The circular layer of visceral musculature exhibits a tonic contraction of sufficient force to close the lumen. The force, however, must be small enough not to compromise blood flow in the tissue. The available evidence indicates that the muscle contracts just enough to shorten the muscle to the required degree without maintaining enough force to raise very much the pressure within the tissue.

Although this tonic shortening force clearly arises from the special properties of the muscle itself, it appears to be regulated, mainly by nerves. An increase in the tone of this sphincter represents the effect of the release of acetylcholine from cholinergic nerves. Such nerves represent the principal, if not the only kind of excitatory motor innervation to this musculature. A reduction in the tone of the sphincter reflects, in all probability, the release of nitric oxide from nitrergic nerves. Such nerves represent the principal, if not the only inhibitory motor nerves to this muscle.

Various factors can alter the activity of such nerves and thus raise the force of contraction in the sphincter. The most important are sensori-motor neural pathways that advance the principal function of the sphincter, the prevention of the return of gastric contents into the esophagus.

The most notable of these pathways involve mechanoreceptors and chemoreceptors in the stomach that can alter sphincter tone in the resting state. These receptors are the endings of sensory nerve fibers that carry nerve impulses to the cell bodies of the motor nerves that supply the sphincteric muscle.

Some hormones can excite the excitatory and inhibitory motor nerves to this sphincter as well as the muscle itself. They were once thought to act importantly in normal physiology. The idea has been largely abandoned because the experimental evidence failed to support it.

The force of the sphincteric tone at rest is sometimes found to be greatly reduced or even eliminated. Such a change counters the essential function of the sphincter to keep the gastric contents out of the esophagus. The physiological basis for a sustained reduction of tone in the esophagogastric sphincter in various pathological states remains to be fully investigated. There are many possible explanations.

5.3.2. The Organ in Action

5.3.2.1. The Esophageal Body

The operation of the esophagus after a swallow is fully as stereotyped as that of the pharynx. Its action begins with the closure of the pharyngoesophageal sphincter (whose operation is described above as a part of the pharynx). The burst of nerve activity that makes that sphincter contract after pharyngeal contraction simply continues into the esophageal body as though it is a single event, one motion.

The impulse to contract contraction then moves as a front along the esophagus toward the stomach, passing with no grossly evident interruption from the sphincter into the esophagus, from the striated muscle segment to the smooth muscle part, and on to the gastric junction. (Actually, a sufficiently detailed and critical analysis of esophageal motions reveals a slight interruption at the striated-smooth muscle junction consistent with the underlying physiological mechanisms, but this delay is insignificant in terms of the fluid-mechanical functions of the organ). The contraction appears to fully occlude the lumen at all points along the organ. Its duration, as measured at a single point, indicates that the moving front of the relaxation that must follow the contraction front lags behind it by several centimeters in man. Thus, the wave length of the esophageal peristaltic contraction is great, 10 centimeters or more. Limitations of methods, however, do not allow this relaxation front to be actually observed very well in man.

Although most observers think only of the circular muscle layer in relation to esophageal motility, the outer longitudinal muscle layer and the parallel mucosal muscle layer also participate in this event. They tend to draw the gastric end of the organ, which is relatively mobile, toward the more firmly fixed pharyngeal end where the parapharyngeal muscles anchor it to the skull. The gastric end of the esophagus, however, cannot be moved enough to pull the stomach very far into the thorax, for the phrenoesophageal ligament anchors the esophagus to the diaphragm. There may be some motion of the esophagus through the esophageal hiatus in the diaphragm, but the ligament must limit this. The shortening of the esophageal body that takes place in swallowing is compensated by an elongation in a short segment of the organ at and just above the esophagogastric sphincter. This part lengthens under the influence of an inhibitory innervation that is activated at the same time that an excitatory innervation is activating the two longitudinal muscle layers. Thus, the esophagogastric junction stays essentially within the diaphragmatic hiatus and its anchoring phrenoesophageal ligament, though stretched a bit, remains intact. The rigidity of the wall created by the axial contraction may facilitate the flow of the swallowed bolus by preventing the expansion of the lumen under the influence of the force exerted by the peristaltic contraction on the bolus.

5.3.2.2. The Esophagogastric Sphincter

The relaxation of the esophagogastric sphincter that occurs in a swallow takes place at about the same time that the pharyngoesophageal sphincter contracts. Thus, the esophageal lumen is open to the stomach for the full duration of the time required for the propulsive esophageal contraction to traverse the esophageal body, a matter of several seconds.

The inhibition of the smooth muscle that is known to precede contraction in the caudal two-thirds of the esophageal body (see below) takes place essentially simultaneously throughout the whole of the organ, including the sphincter. The sphincter remains relaxed for several seconds, its tone returning only when the front of the contraction traveling along the esophageal body reaches it. The front simply moves from the esophageal body into the sphincter and makes the sphincter contract, the force of its contraction rising well above that which characterizes the resting state for a few seconds before it falls back to that level.

5.3.3. The Program of Esophageal Motor Function

The main facts of the program that coordinates these events in swallowing are indisputable, but the details remain to be fully described. The initiation of events takes place in the same brainstem centers that also govern pharyngeal peristalsis. The striated musculature of the esophagus is governed in the same way as that of the pharynx. In contrast, the program that governs the sequence in the visceral muscle of the distal esophagus depends on peripheral mechanisms located in the wall of the organ.

Motor events in both parts of the esophagus are triggered wholly through the tenth cranial (vagus) nerves, with complete bilateral representation in the organ of both the right and left vagal centers. That is to say, the nerve fibers from the two sides of the brainstem are completely mixed because of the amalgamation of the two vagus nerves into the esophageal plexus. The discharge of the tenth nerve (vagal) motor nuclei always follows that of the ninth nerve (glossopharyngeal) nuclei in such a way that the operation of the pharynx and esophagus appears grossly as a smooth and uniform process.

In the striated muscle segment of the esophageal body, as in the pharynx, the progression of the contraction front must represent the serial discharge of motor units in a craniocaudal sequence. A motor unit is a single somatic motor nerve fiber together with the fixed number of striated muscle cells innervated by that fiber, which must contract simultaneously when that fiber discharges. The motor unit in this esophageal musculature is estimated to be a matter of ten cells or so, the size of motor units in the pharynx and fine somatic muscles such as the extraocular muscles. Since the nerve cell bodies for these somatic nerves lie in the vagal nuclei of the brainstem, the program for this progression must be located in the brainstem.

In the smooth muscle segment of the esophageal body, a motor unit organization does not exist. Anatomic evidence shows that a single motor nerve cell spreads its axons over a vast range of muscle tissue and the effective ranges of adjacent motor nerve cell bodies must overlap a great deal. That is to say, there is no fixed relationship between a single nerve fiber and a population of muscle cells.

The progression of the contraction front in the smooth muscle segment depends upon a peripheral program that is, as yet, not completely understood. It is clear that it involves the release of nitric oxide from motor nerves in the myenteric plexus and that the first event in the process is the inhibition of contraction. The visceral muscle cannot express this inhibition mechanically in the normal organ because this smooth muscle has no tone. However, the inhibitory phase can be demonstrated where the muscle is examined in terms of its myoelectrical activity or when it has been made to contract by artificial means. The period of inhibition produced by excitation of the inhibitory nitrergic motor nerves is followed by a contraction. This contraction of the circular muscle is responsible for esophageal peristalsis. Thus, the esophageal peristaltic contraction appears to be a rebound to antecedent inhibition. Some evidence suggests that this rebound contraction also involves the release of acetylcholine from the same motor nerves. The fact that this rebound contraction is delayed longer and longer from the top of the esophageal body to the bottom is unexplained. The general point, however, is that the progression of the contraction front along the smooth muscle part of the esophageal body represents a gradient of unknown nature in the physiology of the neuromuscular relationship rather that a central program or a particular structural arrangement within the intrinsic nerves of the organ.

The relaxation of the lower esophageal sphincter reflects simply the inhibition of the muscle by the nitric oxide-releasing inhibitory nerves of the myenteric plexus. The brief powerful contraction of the sphincter at the end of the relaxation is the same rebound response to inhibition.

The tone that the sphincter exhibits at rest is clearly not neurogenic. It reflects a special biochemical property of that muscle itself, as reflected in special features of its mitochondrial morphology and in the nature of the energy metabolism, characteristics that distinguish it from the visceral muscle of the esophageal body.

The place of the interstitial cells of Cajal of the esophagus in this control system is conjectural. Their geometry suggests that they are interposed between the motor nerves and the smooth muscle of the circular layer and that they serve to make both contractions and relaxations radially symmetrical.

5.3.4. Esophageal Flow

A fluid bolus that passes from the pharynx into the esophagus enters as a little jet, a squirt, and it can move a considerable distance under the propulsive force of the pharyngeal contraction. More viscous boluses can also enter rapidly, getting well ahead of the moving front of the esophageal peristaltic contraction. Undoubtedly, the erect posture used by man and many other primates in eating enhances the movement of such a bolus a long way ahead of the esophageal peristaltic contraction. The force of the pharyngeal squirt combined with hydrostatic force may carry a liquid bolus rapidly, essentially unimpeded, through the flaccid esophagus and esophagogastric sphincter into the stomach. Usually, the bolus is of an intermediate viscosity, and it moves largely under the peristaltic force. A very resistant solid bolus may move only under the force of the esophageal peristaltic contraction. In such a case, it will require several seconds to traverse the esophagus because it takes that long for the peristaltic contraction to move that far. In any case, the bolus slows as it reaches the level of the diaphragm. With the usual swallowed bolus, a material of mixed composition that includes quite solid matter, some solids in the bolus often remain behind the liquid components until the advancing contraction sweeps any residue out of the caudal part of the organ.

The full force of the contraction front can convey solid boluses of considerable size throughout the entire organ. Even very solid things, such as large tablets or coins, are transported to the stomach readily by the esophageal contraction. The distensibility of the organ throughout its entire length allows it to accommodate and pass objects of astonishing diameter.

The saliva provides lubrication that critically facilitates the esophageal transport of solids. This lubricating function of saliva is not its only role in swallowing. Swallowed unconsciously throughout both the day and the night, saliva constantly bathes the esophageal mucosa with a weak buffer solution. This process opposes the erosion of the esophageal mucosa by refluxed gastric acid and pepsin and removes bile salts and any corrosive drugs that may be present in the refluxed contents of the stomach. The importance of this constant bath of saliva to esophageal function becomes clear in disease states where salivary flow in diminished.

5.4. STOMACH AND PYLORIC SPHINCTER

Although the stomach constitutes a set of parts or elements with different modes of operation, these merge into one another one another so cunningly that the complex organ seems to act as a single unit. Anatomical nomenclature designates four elements in the stomach, the gastric fundus, the gastric body, the gastric antrum, and the pylorus (Fig. **3** and Fig. **4**). This essentially structural terminology does not wholly conform to the physiological distinctions that identify the separate functional parts of the stomach. It acts as a unit with two parts, the proximal and distal parts of the stomach, that merge into one another in mechanical terms (Fig. **5**).

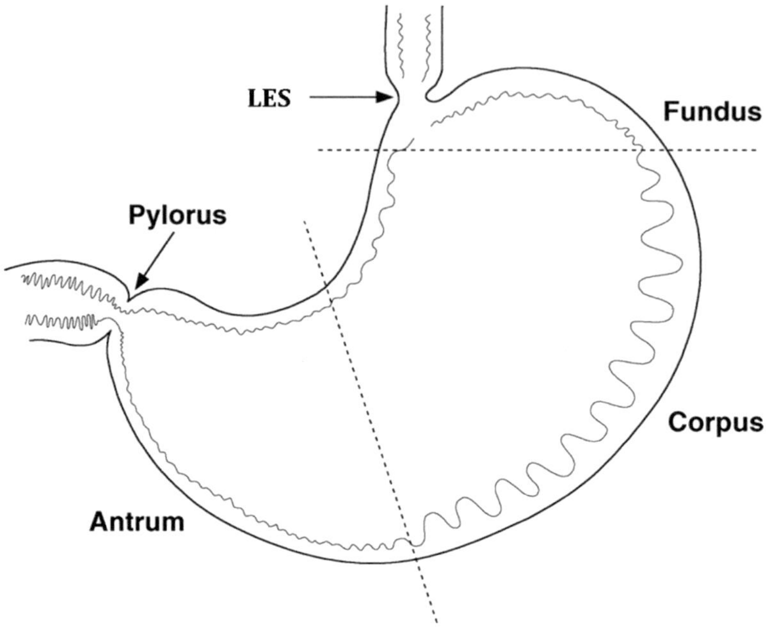

Figure 3: The parts of the human stomach as they are designated in conventional anatomic terminology. These terms do not correlate with the functional elements of the stomach. The two functional regions, proximal (or rostral) and distal (or caudal) merge into one another.

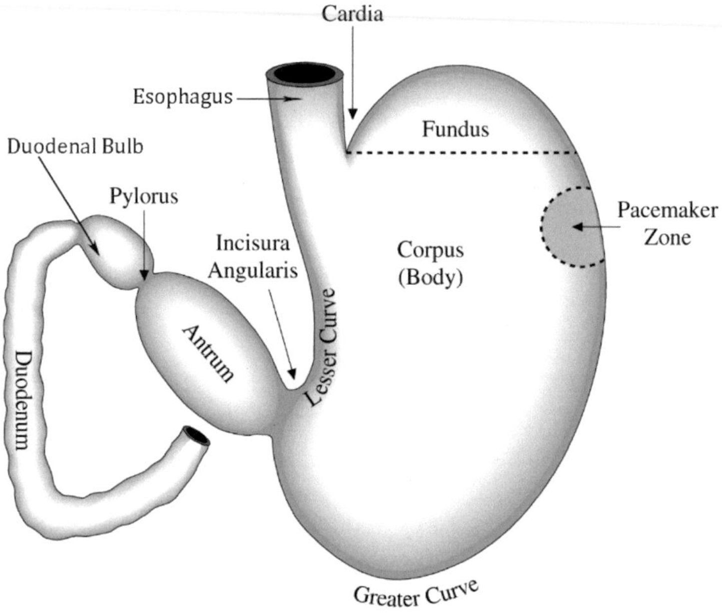

Figure 4: A schematic view of the stomach showing the different regions including the pacesetter region in the proximal part of the stomach.

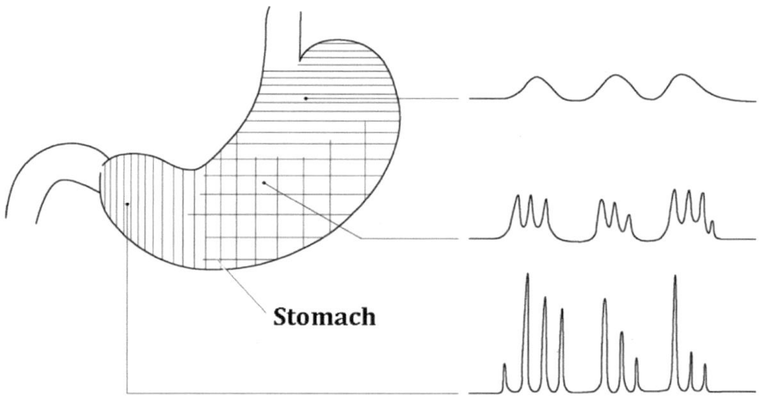

Figure 5: The simultaneous recording of contractions from three levels of the stomach reveal the fact that the three regions differ in the force of the rhythmic contractions that they produce, with a pronounced gradient such that the most powerful activity occurs in the most caudal region.

The fundus, body and antrum are treated here together, as a single anatomical unit, the stomach. The pyloric sphincter, however, is treated as a separate element in the operation of the stomach because of its structural and functional distinctions.

5.4.1. The Organ "at Rest": The Fasted State

5.4.1.1. The Stomach

The stomach never really rests. Instead, it shows two different patterns of contraction that depend on the cycle of eating. These are called, respectively, the "fed" and the "fasted" patterns.

The resting state of the stomach refers to its state in the period after it has emptied itself of ingested matter. That process of emptying may take as long as six hours after a meal. The organ then enters into a particular manner of action, the "fasted pattern" of motility that continues until something is eaten again, whereupon it returns to the "fed pattern" that is characteristic of the fed state.

When it is empty of food, the stomach is quiet for most of the time, rousing to action only at long periods. Both the antrum and the fundus are collapsed. Actually, we know very little for certain about gastric movements in this state because the presence of any significant mass of extrinsic matter in the lumen, such as radiopaque solutions and balloons, makes the stomach, by definition, no longer empty. However, both the pressures measured from thin open-tipped tubes and the electromyogram recorded from wires implanted in the gastric wall probably represent fairly faithfully the active state of the empty stomach, at least the limited part of it that they can reveal. The concepts presented here represent conjectures made from such studies. The results of ultrasonographic studies of the empty stomach support these conjectures.

In the fasted state, the fundus of the stomach is probably completely and continuously inactive. The antrum, however, is not. It periodically arouses from a state of complete inactivity to show the intermittent contractions of antral peristalsis (see below). These build up to a short episode in which the antrum contracts at the maximum possible rate and amplitude. The action then subsides in a moment to a state of torpor, complete inactivity, that continues for about an hour when the intermittent contractions reappear in a crescendo again reaching the climax of maximal activity. This cycle, continuing as long as the fast lasts, was long ago linked to the hunger pangs characteristic of fasting. Such feelings correspond to the climactic burst of maximal activity. This cycling is a part of a more general cyclic activity that involves mainly the small intestine. It is described in more detail in that part of this chapter (see below).

The periodic contractions of the gastric antrum that take place in fasting consist of the movements that characterize antral peristalsis, described in detail in the next section. This periodic activity serves to clear the stomach of fluids, the saliva delivered by the normal and unconscious process of repeated swallowing, and the secretions produced continuously by the gastric mucosa.

We know nothing of the movements of the gastric mucosa in this state. Since gastric secretion continues, it seems likely that the mucosal muscle remains active because mucosal motions may well be critical to assist the flow of secreted gastric juice out of the gastric glands and away from the mucosal surface.

5.4.1.2. The Pyloric Sphincter

The pyloric sphincter always operates in combination with antral peristalsis. Thus, the state of the sphincter at rest corresponds to that of the antrum. When the antrum is inactive, manifesting no rhythmic peristaltic contractions, the pylorus is resting in a stable state in which a moderate degree of tone in its circular muscle layer closes the lumen. When the antrum contracts peristaltically as it does periodically in the migrating motor complex, the pylorus also participates, relaxing with the approach of each peristaltic contraction and contracting when the peristaltic wave reaches it (see below).

5.4.2. The Organ in Action: The Mechanics of Filling and Emptying

5.4.2.1. The Stomach: "Receptive Relaxation"

As soon as the ingestion of food and fluid begins, the periodic activity of the gastric antrum ends and the fundus begins the process called "receptive relaxation". This term refers to the fact that the muscle of the fundus of the stomach relaxes as the stomach fills, allowing the luminal capacity of this part of the organ to increase. This expansion of the volume of the stomach permits intragastric pressure to remain constant over a very large range of volumes. The magnitude of this change is huge, for the full stomach (in man) may hold as much as two liters, while the volume of fluid obtained by aspiration from the "empty" stomach is only 50 ml or less. (True emptiness never occurs in the stomach because its mucosa is always secreting at least a little fluid, the gastric juice). The "empty" stomach is made smaller by the shortening of the fibers of the fundic oblique muscle layer and possibly by collapse of the organ. The thick folds of mucosa present in the empty stomach arise from buckling that must represent a constant intramural tension, possibly arising from active contraction, possibly reflecting residual stress, an intrinsic property of the tissue.

This process of relaxation and elongation of the muscle of the gastric fundus characterizes especially the oblique muscle layer because the increase in volume produces an expansion especially in the fundus, an elongation of the organ in the axis of direction of the fibers of the oblique muscle layer. That layer exists only in the part of the stomach that expands the most. The fundus is three-dimensional, of course, and so some relaxation must occur in the other muscle layers in the fundus as well. The expansion also takes place, to a lesser degree, in the region intermediate between the fundus and the antrum, the part of the stomach called the gastric body. Receptive relaxation appears to involve the antrum comparatively little.

5.4.2.2. The Stomach: Antral Peristalsis

With the ingestion of food, the antrum begins a new type of activity, a stable pattern of contractions called antral peristalsis. Each peristaltic contraction begins as a shallow indentation of the lumen along the lesser curvature at the junction between the fundus and the gastric body. The contraction first forms a shallow ring around the whole viscus. At the same time, it begins to move forward, toward the pylorus, away from the point on the lesser curvature where it first appears. The contraction moves constantly toward the pylorus, accelerating continuously and becoming deeper and broader. As it approaches the pylorus, it becomes fully occlusive of the lumen and comes to occupy the whole length of the antrum. At about the time the contraction is beginning to dissipate at the level of the pylorus, a new one is forming at the starting point on the lesser curvature at the junction between the fundus and the gastric body.

This cycle continues over and over, the period of the peristaltic cycle in man being about twenty seconds or an integral multiple of about twenty seconds. During the time that the stomach contains food, only about half of the twenty-second cycles that are available for an antral peristaltic contraction actually contain such contractions, on average. That is, the average level of peristaltic activity is about half the maximum possible. The antral peristaltic contraction in the fed state seems to be identical to that in the fasted state except that, in the short interludes of maximal activity that take place periodically in fasting, they occur in every available time slot, at twenty-second intervals.

Although the impulse to contract progresses along the antrum from the very the beginning of each peristaltic event, it accelerates so much that, at the end of each event, it appears to be simultaneous at adjacent points along the antrum. For that reason, each peristaltic cycle is said to end in a "terminal antral contraction". That is, the last few centimeters of the antrum appear to contract simultaneously. This terminal antral contraction involves the pylorus, for pyloric contractions and relaxations correlate with the terminal antral contraction and its relaxation.

Clearly, the circular muscle layer is the main player in antral peristalsis. The conspicuous behavior of the pyloric muscle ring is probably mimicked by the other loop of the double torus formed by this muscle (see chapter I), but the other (more rostral) loop of the torus cannot be seen very clearly most of the time at gross inspection of the organ. Nevertheless, a slight indentation of the antrum, commonly present at the position of that loop, reveals its contraction as being a little stronger than that of the adjacent antral muscle. The contraction of this secondary loop of the pyloric torus may sometimes be seen to form a partial occlusion at the top of the antrum. It is likely that the drawing together of these two conjoined loops of the pyloric torus serves to shorten the antrum during the terminal antral contraction. The contraction of the outer longitudinal muscle layer in the antrum probably does so as well. Such shortening of the antrum in antral peristalsis is visually apparent but it has not been adequately analyzed.

5.4.2.3. The Pyloric Sphincter

The pyloric sphincter always operates as though it is a part of the antrum. It differs from the antrum only in its capacity to maintain a stable tonic contraction.

Thus, when the terminal part of the antrum is not in a contracted state, as at the initiation of a peristaltic contraction in the body of the stomach, the pylorus maintains the closure of the lumen at the gastroduodenal junction by maintaining a stable degree of contraction. As an antral peristaltic contraction approaches the pylorus, the pylorus relaxes. It seems to do so as a part of a front of relaxation that precedes the moving front of the antral contraction. This pyloric relaxation begins at about the same time that the peristaltic contraction enters the antrum. When the front of the peristaltic contraction reaches the level of the pylorus, the sphincter contracts forcefully, the force greatly exceeding that of the tone that normally closes the junction. The force then rapidly declines to the stable tonic force of the pylorus that occludes the lumen at rest.

5.4.3. The Program that Governs Gastric Filling and Emptying

5.4.3.1. The Stomach

The expansion of the fundus that occurs in receptive relaxation seems to be chiefly the result of the action of an inhibitory innervation. The responsible nerves seem to be the same kind as those that relax the esophagogastric sphincter in swallowing, in which nitric oxide is the principal neurohumoral transmitter. This sort of nerve innervates all three layers of muscle in the fundus. It appears to enter the stomach as a part of the craniosacral innervation, passing from the vagus nerves into the esophagus and then through the cardia into the stomach where it is distributed mainly to the fundus.

It is not clear exactly what excites this inhibitory nitrergic innervation to relax the fundus during the process of eating. The possibilities include psychic inputs to vagal centers in the brainstem, inputs from the mouth and chewing apparatus, and inputs from the esophagus. Sensori-motor reflex pathways that are excited by gastric mechanoreceptors also induce such relaxation. These gastric mechanoreceptors are located in the wall of the stomach itself. Some of the reflex pathways are local, involving only the neural structures of the gastric wall. Others are long reflexes that involve vagal centers and outflows.

Antral peristalsis appears to be initiated and sustained by the discharge of excitatory motor nerves, mainly cholinergic nerves (acting through the release of acetylcholine). These also traverse the vagus nerves, reaching the antrum through the gastric branches of the vagal trunks. These excitatory motor nerves trigger the onset of antral peristalsis, their level of activity determining the probability of occurrence of antral peristalsis.

The progressive nature of antral peristalsis, however, is determined not by nerves but by an intrinsic "clock" in the wall of the stomach, an electrical discharge that probably arises in the network of interstitial cells of Cajal in the antrum and passes from that network into the antral musculature. These signals, generically called the electrical slow waves (or the basic electrical rhythm), arise at a pacemaking site on the greater curvature at the top of the antrum and pass, with acceleration and augmentation, toward the pylorus, a new electrical signal appearing at intervals of twenty seconds in man. The new cycle begins just as the former one reaches the pylorus. The signal thus mimics the antral peristaltic contraction in such a way as to reveal itself as the pacemaker for that peristaltic contractile phenomenon. The pacemaker continues at a constant rate while the antral musculature may respond to all cycles, to none, or to any as an intermittent sequence of contractions with an underlying fundamental frequency, under the influence of the excitatory and inhibitory innervation and, perhaps, hormones.

5.4.3.2. The Pyloric Sphincter

The behavior that distinguishes the sphincter from the antrum is its capacity to maintain a tonic contraction at rest. This tone appears to be the consequence of a specialization in the musculature much like that in the musculature of the lower esophageal sphincter.

5.4.4. Gastric Flow

In gastric filling, the material that enters the stomach may contain both liquids and solid masses of disparate consistencies. The stomach must manage the liquids and solids that it receives in quite different ways, for it passes its contents on to the duodenum as a homogeneous fluid of uniform physical consistency.

Swallowed solids are retained at first in the proximal part of the organ, tending to form layers on the wall such that the first layer lies next to the mucosa, with succeeding solids forming in a series of layers inside that. A part of a liquid bolus first coats the innermost solid layer that it encounters, but a greater part of the liquid bolus flows straightaway antegrade into the antrum. Thus, with a meal, solids accumulate as a layered mass in the expanding fundus while the antrum fills with liquids.

In the antrum, each antral peristaltic contraction pushes toward the pylorus a quantum of liquid containing suspended masses or particles of solids. A large fraction of the liquid passes on into the duodenum, as do those solid particles that are small enough. The solid masses that are too large to enter the narrowing lumen are rejected, however, and so they return toward the fundus in a motion called retropulsion (Fig. **6**). Then they are caught by the next advancing wave of peristaltic contraction to go through the same cycle of propulsion-retropulsion. With each such cycle, the floating solid masses are broken up or dissolved until they are reduced to particles that are small enough to pass into the duodenum. The critical diameter of a mass or particle is about two millimeters or less. This process is referred to as the grinding function of the antrum, or trituration. Thus, the stomach empties in squirts, each jet consisting of liquid containing suspended solid particles of that diameter or less.

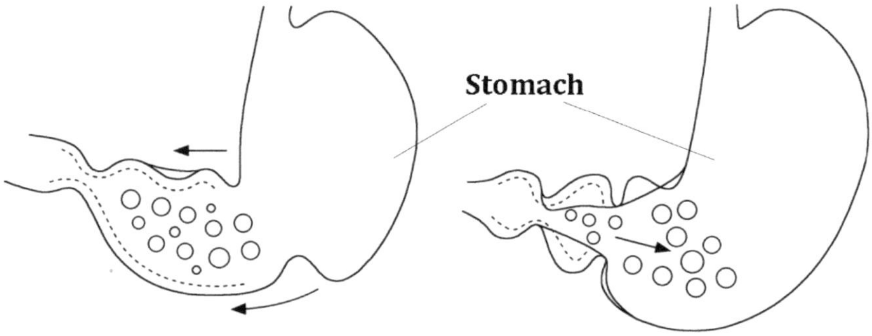

Figure 6: Retropulsion in the stomach. To the left, a diagram shows food particles of various sizes approaching the pylorus together under the influence of a peristaltic contraction (nonocclusive, at this point) that begins to move slowly through the caudal part of the stomach. To the right, the depth and velocity of the accelerating and deepening contraction have selected out the larger particles that are, accordingly, rejected to be picked up by the next peristaltic wave. In this way particles are recycled in a process that is vigorous enough to help break them up as they are softened by digestive enzymes. Thus, only particles less than about 2 mm in diameter reach the duodenum.

A good deal of retrograde flow occurs normally through the pylorus but it is small and inconstant. The determining or controlling factors in retrograde flow remain to be investigated. High degrees of retrograde flow may be important in disease, for bile clearly damages the epithelium of the stomach and esophagus.

The antrum was once said to be the pump (a peristaltic pump) that empties the stomach while the fundus is a simple reservoir. That was the view until only a few years ago. Now, we recognize that the peristaltic activity of the caudal part of the organ alone does not account fully for the pattern of gastric emptying. Much of the force that drives gastric emptying comes from the gradual restoration of the tone of the fundic musculature. A slow and steady rise in this fundic tone presses the solid or plastic fundic content into the antrum which mixes and grinds it and delivers it to the intestine in quanta. Thus, the whole stomach is involved in the process of emptying, the fundus slowly feeding material to the antrum, which does the job of mixing and grinding.

The organ is governed in such a way that the emptying of a liquid meal is exponential. A meal of solids empties more slowly, of course. The time required for a meal to empty is rarely less than roughly two hours, but the time varies greatly with the composition of the meal. Fats delay gastric emptying. The degree of inhibition varies with both the concentration of fat in the meal and the particular fatty acids in the fat. A chemoreceptive reflex mediates this inhibition, the receptors being located in the duodenal epithelium, apparently.

There is some evidence for a degree of antroduodenal coordination. That is, sometimes the arrival of an antral peristaltic contraction at the pylorus seems to enhance the immediate onset of a peristaltic contraction in the most rostral part of the duodenum. This is far from a one-to-one correlation, and, in any case, its significance remains debatable.

5.5. SMALL INTESTINES AND ILEOCECAL SPHINCTER

5.5.1. The Organ at Rest: The Fasted State

The intestine, like the stomach, does not actually rest during a period of fasting but, instead, shows a cyclic pattern of activity resembling that of the gastric antrum. When mechanical activity is recorded at any one point along the intestine in the fasted animal, it alternates from complete inactivity to the maximal activity possible (Fig. 7). This cycle has a long and variable period, often an hour or more.

The most conspicuous event in this cycle (called Phase III) is a short interval (5-10 minutes) of maximal activity in which the contraction occur with maximal force at maximal frequency. This period ends abruptly when a longer period of inactivity (Phase I) begins. It continues for 10-20 minutes. Then, a period (Phase II) characterized by intermittent brief contractions begins They become somewhat more frequent and powerful, culminating in the 5-10 minute period of maximal contractions, Phase III, once more. The length of the period and of its components varies greatly in the individual over time and among members of a group, but the cycling continues as long as the fast lasts. These three phases of the cycle are commonly referred to as Phases I, II and III, Phase I being the period of inactivity, Phase II the longer period of intermittent activity, and Phase III the shortest period, that of maximal activity. The whole pattern is called the "migrating motor complex" (MMC).

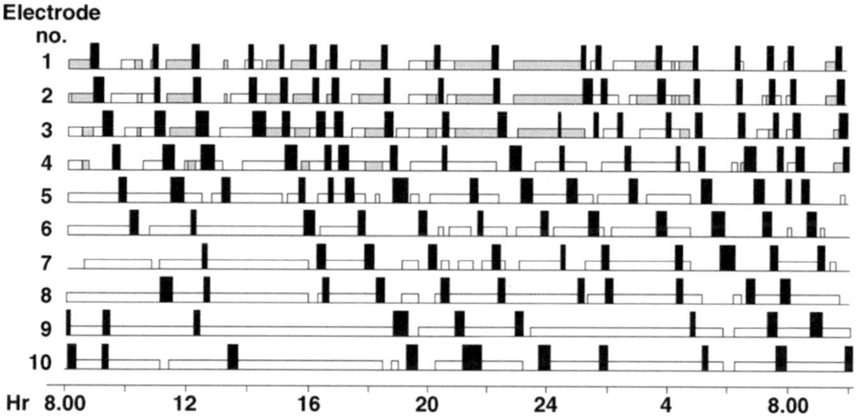

Figure 7: A diagram of the Migrating Motor Complex (MMC), the cyclic variations in motor activity of the small intestine that take place in fasting. The diagram shows 10 traces of the electrical activity that accompany contractions in visceral muscle (spikes, or action potentials) as made from 10 electrodes chronically implanted at uniform intervals along the intestine of an unanesthetized and ambulant experimental animal. The horizontal axis shows time, in hours, for a term of 24 hours. The tall black bars represent the short periods of Phase III, the episodes in which contractions occur with maximal frequency and force. The lower open bars represent the longer periods of Phase II activity in which contractions of less magnitude occur in short bursts or as intermittent repeated events. The parts of the lines without bars represent Phase I, the periods when no contractions occur. The 10 traces together show the fact that the whole phenomenon migrates slowly in the rostrocaudal direction, slowing a little as it approaches the colon. Also, the variability of the cycle is apparent. This same cycling is evident in the stomach, each cycle seeming to begin in the antrum and progress into the intestine.

Within Phase III, the brief period of maximal activity, contractions occur with a highly regular frequency at nearly 12 per minute in the duodenum, declining in steps to about 7 per minute in the ileum. Records taken from a series of closely spaced points reveal that these contractions migrate tens of centimeters caudad at a constant velocity.

When activity is recorded from a series of points along the organ, the whole cycle of the MMC can be seen to occur with a phase lag such that the whole phenomenon appears to move caudad along the intestine. The term "migrating motor complex" (MMC) refers to this property.

The MMC actually begins in the stomach and traverses the small intestine. It does not pass into the large intestine. Its effect appears in the secretion of the pancreas as well, where a brief peak in the volume of secretion accompanies phase III in the intestine. Although the phenomenon involves most conspicuously the phasic contractions of the circular muscle layer of the intestine, the underlying tone of that muscle layer also changes in a cyclic pattern with the MMC, and the longitudinal muscle layer may participate as well. Tone in the circular muscle layer is highest in Phase I, when, presumably flow volume is at its lowest. The mucosal compression produced by tonic contraction of the circular muscle layer must influence mucosal functions, but the effects remain to be studied.

5.5.2. The Organ in Action: Intestinal Mixing and Propulsion after Feeding

With feeding, the activity of the small intestine immediately undergoes a profound and immediate change like that which takes place in the stomach. The cycling pattern of the MMC ends, to be replaced with a pattern of activity in which contractions of the circular muscle layer occur apparently at random in time and space. Being controlled by a pacemaker, they are not actually random but they appear to be so to the uninformed eye.

Recordings made at a single point show that these contractions occur every five seconds or at an integral multiple of five seconds (10, 15, 20...seconds), betraying the effect of an underlying "clock", running continuously. This "clock", of course, runs in the fasted animal as well, and the cycling of the MMC does not influence it. It is the response to the clock, the muscle contraction, which varies cyclically in the MMC. In the fed state, recordings of contractions made at multiple closely spaced loci show that contractions migrate over variable distances of centimeters to tens of centimeters. The clock governs the frequency, the velocity, and the direction of spread of peristaltic contractions.

The level of motor activity in the fed state seems to be about the same all along the intestine except that the fundamental 5-seconds period of the underlying clock increases incrementally along the intestine to about 9 seconds at the end of the ileum. The average level of activity seems to vary little over time so long as the digestive process continues. In general, intestinal contractions occur at about one-third of the maximal possible number over time in the fed state.

Food enters the intestine from the stomach slowly and it traverses the intestine slowly so that the organ contains nutrient matter for about four to six hours after a meal. The pattern of contractions in the intestine continues essentially unchanged throughout this long period. The cyclic pattern that characterizes fasting resumes about four hours after the last meal.

The actions of the circular muscle layer clearly dominate in records made of mechanical events in the intestine, but the longitudinal muscle layer participates as well. It is not clear how the activity of this layer affects or contributes to the records made of intestinal motor function. Events in the longitudinal muscle layer are difficult to study separately from those of the circular layer and so much less is known about them. For example, the spatial and temporal dimensions of contractions in the longitudinal muscle layer remain to be defined, and their timing with respect to those of the circular muscle layer is not accurately known.

The muscle of the mucosa in the intestine must also participate in the mixing and propulsion of the intestinal content but almost nothing is known about this matter. The only studies that have been made (many decades ago) indicate that the mucosal muscle layer can move the mucosa about in various directions, as indicated by the orientation of the muscle fibers. Also, the slips of muscle that extend from the muscularis mucosae into the core of each mucosal villus of the mucosa are able to contract independently. The villi contract individually with pumping movements, each villus shortening rapidly and then re-expanding slowly. The villi can also be seen to move laterally in waves, in a pattern that resembles the waves created by the wind as it passes over a field of wheat. Such movements obviously affect intestinal absorption. They remain to be studied quantitatively and their controls remain unknown.

5.5.3. The Program for Intestinal Mixing and Propulsion

The musculature itself contains the program for the rhythmicity of contractions in the two layers of muscle of the main muscle coat (Fig. **8**). Actually, the program centers in the planar network of interstitial cells of Cajal embedded in the circular layer. Electrodes spaced along the intestine detect the electrical pacemaker, the electrical slow wave or basic electrical rhythm of the intestine, resembling that found in the gastric antrum. The clock in the intestine, however, possesses a higher frequency.

As in the antrum, the electrical slow wave moves essentially as a ring rostrocaudally along the intestine and the contraction, being locked in phase to the electrical signal, must follow it. As the signal passes any point along the intestine, the muscle at that point may choose to contract or not to contract with each cycle of the clock. In the fed state, the muscle contracts in about one-third to one-half of the opportunities, in a quasi-random choice. In the silent phase (Phase I) of the cyclic activity of fasting, the MMC, it responds to none. In the maximal phase of the MMC (Phase III) it contracts to all of them.

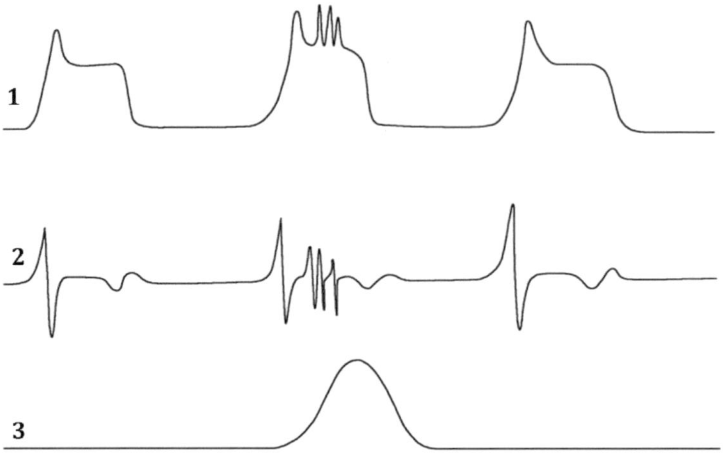

Figure 8: A diagram to show the correlation between electrical activity and contraction in the muscular layers of the intestinal wall. The horizontal axis shows time. The tracing at the top (1) represents the recording of the electrical potential difference across the membrane of a single muscle cell as recorded from a single electrode inserted into the cell. It shows three signals occurring in a temporal sequence and having a uniform basic configuration with an initial spike followed by a plateau. The second tracing from the top (2) represents the same three signals as they would appear in a record made from an electrode applied to the muscle mass, contacting hundreds or thousands of cells at once. It shows the same three signals, although the form is a little different. This indicates that the signals occur throughout all the cells in the muscle mass simultaneously. The bottom trace (3), representing the tension in the muscle mass, shows a contraction in conjunction with the second signal. Observe that the signal accompanying this contraction contains a burst of rapid spikes on the plateau that signal the onset of the contraction. A spike burst can occur only on the plateau of the slow wave. The three recurring signals with an initial spike and a following plateau are slow waves, the units of the basic electrical rhythm, the output of the clock that underlies rhythmic contractions in the intestine. The spike burst on the second of the three signals is an action potential, the electrical equivalent of a contraction.

Each slow wave signal moves antegrade along the intestine as a ring, being simultaneous along the circumference. Since the signal determines the position of the spike burst and since the spike burst determines the position of the contraction, the basic electrical rhythm of the intestine governs the frequency, velocity and direction of spread of peristaltic contractions.

In the human duodenum, the slow waves occur with a period of about 5 seconds. Thus, at any single point, a peristaltic contraction can occur only at integral multiples of 5 seconds, at 5, 10, 15, and 20... seconds.

The rate of the intestinal clock is very stable. It changes only with metabolic rate and body temperature, both of which normally vary over a very narrow range. (Almost certainly, the rates of discharge of the other gastrointestinal pacemakers, in the stomach and large intestine, similarly change with metabolic rate and body temperature). Because of the constant migration of the electrical slow wave downstream along the intestine, the contractions must follow it. In this way, the electrical slow wave regulates both the frequency and the direction of movement of the rhythmic contractions of the intestine.

At any single point along the intestine, a series of slow wave cycles offers a sequence of opportunities for contraction. These opportunities occur at stable intervals, 5 seconds in the human duodenum for example (Fig. **9**).

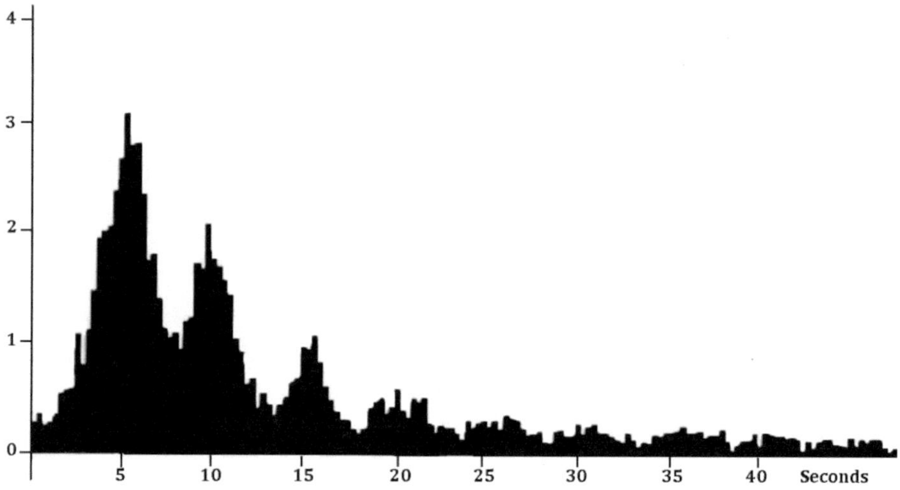

Figure 9: A diagram of the time intervals separating contractions occurring at a single point in the duodenum as recorded from the pressure in a tiny balloon placed in the middle of the organ in fasted ambulant men. The intervals between 7572 successive contractions were measured and plotted here as the number of intervals over the duration of intervals. The stable period of the basic electrical rhythm (electrical slow waves), 5 seconds, is reflected in the fact that the peaks in the frequency histogram occur at 5, 10, 15 and 20 seconds, and so on. The blurring between the peaks could reflect such variables as variation in the period of the clock over time, shifts in the position of the balloon, or artificial pressure peaks induced by body movements such as respiration.

Whether or not a contraction takes place depends especially upon the activity of the motor nerves that supply the muscle. Two principal kinds of motor nerves simultaneously bear upon the intestinal muscle, excitatory and inhibitory nerves. The excitatory neurohormonal transmitter, acetylcholine, and the inhibitory transmitter, nitric oxide, are probably released continuously together in this muscle, the net effects of their action being expressed not necessarily as an arithmetic summation but rather in the form of some more complicated interaction between the two at the neuromuscular interface. They have vastly different characteristics as transmitters in, for example, the rate of synthesis, the rate of release, the duration of effect, the rate of degradation, the mechanism of action on the receptors of the muscle cell membrane, *etc*. The nature of their interaction at the neuromuscular interface remains unknown. Actually, nerve fibers in intestinal muscle contain several potential neurotransmitters co-localized in the same terminals and presumably released together with nerve excitation. This fact makes it impossible to assign a single transmitter the full responsibility for any effect produced by nerve stimulation.

Contractions are graded in force. The mechanism of this gradation probably also involves variation in the balance between opposing neural influences on the muscle.

The regulation of the cycling of gastrointestinal motor activity, the MMC, seen in the fasting state seems to reflect the effect of a cycling phenomenon in the central nervous system that is transmitted to the gut both through its external innervation and through the release of hormones. It remains to be investigated more fully.

Early students of intestinal motility credited the Bayliss-Starling reflex (the "Law of the Intestine") for the antegrade propulsion of intestinal contents. For decades, it was considered to account fully for the rostrocaudal transport along the intestine. In this reflex, the stretch of the intestinal wall incites a contraction above (rostral to) the point of stretch and inhibition of contraction below (caudal to) it. The anatomical and physiological evidence for such a reflex does not necessarily establish it as the major mechanism in normal intestinal propulsion. Two obvious facts call the idea into question. First, in its normal function the intestine seems to be rarely, if ever, stretched to the degree needed to excite the reflex. Second, if the reflex were the whole and sufficient mechanism, propulsion along the intestine would occur much faster than it does, by about an order of magnitude. The Bayliss-Starling reflex may well exist only to operate in exceptional circumstances, when the intestine is distended by a potentially obstructing mass. However, it seems obvious that such a reflex would have to be oriented in such a way as to foster antegrade flow rather than retrograde flow.

The program for the movement of the intestinal mucosal muscle can only be surmised, for we lack a ready means to look at that musculature in the living animal. The only thing that seems to be likely is the participation of the submucosal plexus of nerves in the regulation of this musculature. The fact that this intramural plexus is vastly better developed in the small intestine than it is anywhere else in the gastrointestinal tract indicates its importance in the processes of nutrient absorption, for that is the principal function of that organ. That is, the muscle of the mucosa in the intestine is probably critical in the optimization of absorption, and so it makes sense that its movements must be complex. The submucosal plexus governs those motions and so that muscle should require an especially complex and dense innervation.

5.5.4. Small Intestinal Flow

Both the anatomical and behavioral complexity of the small intestine prevent a detailed analysis of the flow of its contents by direct observation. The only direct method, the radiographic observation of radiopaque materials, is severely limited not only by the geometry and the complexity of intestinal movements but also by the unavoidably foreign nature of the observed materials, usually fluids mixed with barium sulfate. These are much denser than any normal foods, and they are unabsorbed. Thus, the usual radiographic studies of intestinal flow examine the organ after it has fasted for a long time (when its behavior is varying widely as it does in the MMC), and it deals with a substrate in which nothing is digested and from which nothing is absorbed and whose volume does not change as it passes through the organ. These study conditions seem very far from normal. Also, the time constraints of exposure to ionizing radiation in man make extensive study by such techniques impossible. Thus, any analysis of intestinal flow by such radiographic means must be capable of indicating, qualitatively or approximately, only the grossest aspects of flow. Such direct study shows that net flow is antegrade, that a large amount of retrograde flow occurs transiently, that there is a great deal of mixing, and that the time required for the intestine to empty itself varies a great deal.

Numerical simulation, a technique that has been applied to intestinal flow only very tentatively, indicates that the advancing front of annular contraction of the circular muscle layer in peristalsis, a moving ring-contraction, causes essentially unidirectional movement of the luminal fluid with comparatively little transfer between the periphery of the cylindrical conduit and the core. Such modeling also indicates that the moving front of contraction in the longitudinal muscle layer (a moving sleeve-contraction) must cause considerable interchange of material between the periphery and the core of the lumen.

Modeling has not taken into account the convolutions of the mucosa in contractions. Obviously, the concurrence of repeated rhythmic contractions in all three muscle layers must lead to complex flows indeed. It should be noted that the rates of movement in the contractions of the muscle layers are so slow that mixing flows must be wholly laminar.

The absorption of nutrient materials, the principal function of the intestine, constitutes the flux of rather simple molecules across a semipermeable membrane, the apical membrane of the intestinal epithelial cell. The process depends in some cases on the ordinary diffusion of molecules across the epithelium and in other cases on the energy-dependent transfer of certain molecules by enzymatic processes located within the epithelial cell membrane, commonly referred to as membrane pumps. Such a process, called active transport, accomplishes the absorption of many simple carbohydrates and amino acids.

These pumps, of course, can transfer nutrients only as fast as they receive them at the luminal surface. Consequently, the rate of absorption, in all cases, is limited by the rate at which these molecules reach the epithelial surface under the influence of the circulation of the fluid within the lumen. Since there is always an unstirred layer of luminal fluid at the mucosal surface through which the molecules must diffuse, the thickness of that layer must be the critical step in absorption. The reduction of this unstirred layer to a minimum seems, on simple inferential grounds, to be the reason for the motions of the mucosal muscle in the intestine. As mentioned above, the villi have been seen to exhibit several kinds of motions, including pumping movements. The way in which such villous motility influences fluid flow across the luminal surface remains an untouched problem that is probably amenable to investigation only by mathematical modeling methods.

5.6. THE BILIARY TRACT AND GALLBLADDER

The motor function of the biliary tract regulates the delivery of bile and pancreatic juice to the duodenum. Since these fluids critically participate in digestion, the enzymatic reduction of the complex substances in foods to the small molecules that can be absorbed, the delivery of these fluids must be closely correlated with eating and the consequent delivery of nutrient material to the duodenum from the stomach.

The force of the contractions of the sparse musculature of the biliary tract is so small that it cannot be reliably measured by direct means. Our ideas about this activity come from experiments in which the flow patterns are visually evaluated and in which pressures are measured. Accordingly, there is almost nothing that can be said quantitatively or precisely about the force and timing contractions of biliary tract muscle. We can only infer the motions of the muscular structures from what is seen in the way the fluids flow through the system.

The production of bile and pancreatic juice never really ceases completely but continues throughout a fast of the duration that occurs in a pattern of normal eating. Both fluids flow down their respective ducts, but at a comparatively low rate. The pancreatic fluid simply escapes into the duodenum through the incompetent sphincter. The bile, in contrast, is diverted, a fraction (about one-third to one-half the volume on average over time) flowing into the common bile duct and into the duodenum and the remainder passing through the cystic duct into the gallbladder.

This diversion of bile into the gallbladder seems to reflect a resistance to flow through the sphincter such that intrabiliary pressure is maintained at a high enough level to overcome the resistance offered by the cystic duct and the contracted gallbladder. The resistance to flow through the sphincter represents, probably, a degree of tonic contraction of this muscle as well as the shutting off of the peristaltic pump that is contained in the sphincter. There could well be some active relaxation of the gallbladder muscle as well to encourage the filling of the gallbladder, but that is not established.

With the ingestion of a meal, hormones released from the gastrointestinal tract stimulate the liver and pancreas to increase greatly the rate of production of the fluids they make. Flow into the ductular system correspondingly increases. The resistance to flow in the sphincter falls, enhancing flow of bile and pancreatic juice into the duodenum. There may also be activation of the peristaltic pump that lies in the sphincter. The gallbladder muscle contracts very slowly in a tonic contraction, expressing its concentrated bile. The volume of bile it contains declines very slowly, so that after one hour about one-third of the volume contained in the organ still remains there. It seems likely that the gallbladder never approaches a state of emptiness, the filling that characterizes the fasting state beginning again before the volume at the onset of the meal has been more or less completely expelled.

Conventional teaching gives the gastrointestinal hormones all the responsibility for the coordination of contractions in the biliary tract. In this scheme, peptide hormones, such as gastrin and cholecystokinin, are released from the gastrointestinal tract to circulate in the blood stream and so reach sensitive receptors in the muscles and nerves of the biliary tract. According to this idea, the muscle of the sphincter responds reciprocally to the muscle of the gallbladder, the sphincter relaxing when the gallbladder is contracting. So deeply entrenched is this scheme that no real alternative or more thoroughly elaborated hypothesis has been proposed. The theory gives little role to the innervation known to exist in this musculature. It does not incorporate an explanation for the regulation of the peristaltic pump that has been demonstrated in the sphincter of Oddi.

5.7. THE LARGE INTESTINE (OR COLON) AND ANAL SPHINCTER

The mammalian large intestine, which includes the internal anal sphincter and, functionally, the external anal sphincter, serves three general functions

- It removes water from the gastrointestinal content
- It allows bacteria to degrade undigested carbohydrate components of the luminal fluid so that the products of digestion can be absorbed by the colonic epithelium, and
- It regulates the exit of the residue of digestion and absorption

The first function relates the adaptation of animals to a terrestrial environment. Thus, the large intestine becomes a large or conspicuous organ only in terrestrial animals. It is comparatively rudimentary in fish and amphibia but more completely developed in the Reptilia.

The second function makes for the more efficient use of foodstuffs. Thus, among the carnivorous mammals and marsupials, the large intestine is structurally comparatively simple because the digestion of meat is largely complete in the small intestine so that the mass of undigested residue that proceeds into the large intestine is comparatively small and contains relatively little nutrient matter. In contrast to meats, the digestion of complex carbohydrates is not complete in the small intestine in any animal. Herbivorous mammals and marsupials thus possess a larger and more complex large intestine to allow for the intracolonic bacterial degradation of such undigested food material into absorbable molecules. This is a mechanism for increased nutritional efficiency.

The third function of the large intestine seems likely to be related to the need for marking territory in the predation that takes place among wild animals. Many predatory species seem to defecate in specific places in relation to hunting or domestic territories. Also, the targets of predators may well need to have the capacity to regulate their defecation partly as a means to evade predation.

Much less can be said with confidence about the motor operation of the large intestine than can be said about that of the rest of the alimentary canal. The organ is poorly accessible, complex, unstable, and unpleasant. It form varies among animals more than the form of any other organ. Our current concepts, outlined below, come from the use of many different methods, all of them having severe limitations, in many kinds of animals. Thus, the global account given here is necessarily highly inferential.

5.7.1. The Organ "at Rest"

Unlike the other organs of the gastrointestinal tract, the large intestine rests during sleep regardless of the condition of feeding or fasting. The available evidence indicates the absence of any sort of rhythmic activity in the large intestine during sleep. The internal anal sphincter remains closed in sleep by a tonic contraction. Rhythmic contractions of the whole organ reappear almost instantly on awakening. Thus, the activity of this organ seems to be much more clearly related to events in the central nervous system than are the motor events of the other viscera.

It is not at all clear how this selectivity in respect to sleep is accomplished. It could be related to the distinctive craniosacral innervation of the large intestine. That component of the extrinsic innervation of the large intestine occurs principally through the sacral part of the craniosacral outflow, whereas the cranial component dominates the more rostral parts of the alimentary canal. Yet sleep represents neurological process in the brain, not in the sacral cord!

5.7.2. The Organ in Action: Water Extraction and Defecation

During waking hours, the large intestine maintains a somewhat variable level of motor activity, its contractions peaking briefly after eating. Actually, there are two brief peaks in activity after a meal, one that begins within a few minutes, and a second that occurs a little later, after some tens of minutes.

The organ is never wholly empty except after vigorous purgation, and so its motor activity should not vary much with the state of feeding or fasting. Its activity has been seen to vary to some degree, however, in some experimental animals. After a prolonged fast, the level of activity fluctuates periodically but much less intensely than it does in the small intestine and with a quite different period from that of the MMC.

The geometry of the contractions in the large intestine remains to be fully described. However, it is clear that the organ constitutes effectively three organs in series, each showing a somewhat different pattern of motor activity.

Throughout the longest part of the organ, the segment between the hepatic flexure and the rectosigmoid junction, the circular muscle layer exhibits a high degree of tone in bands of muscle separated by a few centimeters. These bands appear as rings of constrictions, the "haustral markings" that partially occlude the lumen. They have this name because they seem to divide the organ into a series of pockets called haustra (from the Greek word for the buckets of a water wheel). These serial constrictions occupy most of the length of this part of the organ for most of the time, while the circular muscle layer between these tonically contracted bands seems to be fully relaxed. These contracted bands remain stationary; that is, they show no tendency to migrate in either rostral or caudal directions. From time to time, however, they disappear, the tone of the haustral contractions apparently falling abruptly over a long section of this segment of the intestine. This event is followed by a peristaltic contraction, a ring contraction that moves quite rapidly through the section where the tone has diminished. This is the so-called "mass movement" of the large intestine.

The part of the organ rostral to the hepatic flexure shows a different pattern of activity. Here, stationary indentations due to rings of tonic contraction, the haustral markings, are shallow to absent. Instead, shallow peristaltic ring contractions originate near the hepatic flexure and migrate toward the cecal apex. They are called, for that reason, antiperistaltic contractions. They seem to be excited by the entry of material into the cecum. They are not immutably antiperistaltic: at intervals they become orthoperistaltic, moving from the cecal tip toward the hepatic flexure.

The part of the organ caudal to the rectosigmoid junction, the region commonly called the rectum, exhibits no haustral markings at all. Peristaltic contractions occur in the rectum only at long intervals as a part of the complex movements that occur in defecation. Normal defecation calls forth a single powerful peristaltic contraction that traverses the entire rectosigmoid part of the large intestine.

The internal anal sphincter shows a reasonably stable tonic contraction at rest that is sufficient to fully occlude the lumen. This tonic contraction disappears as the first event in the initiation of defecation and returns only after the rectum has emptied. It is constantly present otherwise, apparently, though it seems to undergo changes in the magnitude of the force of contraction. The factors responsible for such variation remain to be adequately studied.

In defecation, the tone of the internal anal sphincter disappears as the first event, an involuntary phenomenon. This seems to occur quite gradually, rather that as a sudden event. The voluntary contraction of the external anal sphincter (a somatic muscle that surrounds the anal opening in the pelvic floor) can be contracted voluntarily to maintain continence. A peristaltic contraction that fully occludes the lumen begins at some point in the large intestine rostral to the rectum and sweeps slowly throughout the segment, all the way to the internal anal sphincter. This, of course, expels the contents of the rectum. After the rectum has been emptied, the tone of the internal anal sphincter is restored.

5.7.3. The Program for Water Extraction and for Defecation

Just as in the small intestine, the program for the mechanical processes in the large intestine that accomplish the extraction of water from the fecal volume lies principally within the muscle mass and seems to be seated mainly in the plexus of interstitial cells of Cajal. In the large intestine, the planar network of interstitial cells of Cajal lies on the inner (or luminal) surface of the circular muscle layer, forming a floor, as it were, for the submucosa. Electrodes spaced along this surface reveal the presence here of a pacemaker very much like that of the stomach and small intestine, the electrical slow wave or basic electrical rhythm, but running at a slower frequency. It arises in this plane of interstitial cells of Cajal on the inner surface of the circular muscle layer.

As in the small intestine, this signal moves essentially as a ring along the organ, but the pattern of its spread differs from that in the small intestine. For much of the time, the signal moves from a point at about the hepatic flexure toward the cecal apex, while, at the same time, the same signal sends a mirror image in the opposite direction toward the rectum. The retrograde movement of the electrical slow waves in the rostral part of the large intestine is not fixed. From time to time, under the control of unknown factors, the signals reverse, originating at the cecal apex and sweeping downstream. The electrical slow wave signals diminish in magnitude as they move toward the rectosigmoid part of the large intestine. The rectum possesses no detectable slow waves.

Each slow wave may trigger a contraction or it may not. When a contraction occurs, it must follow the signal, the signal governing both its direction and its velocity. Thus, peristaltic contractions in the large intestine arise from the same mechanism as those in the small intestine, differing only quantitatively.

The likelihood of the muscle to respond to an electrical signal with a contraction is much lower in the large intestine than it is in the intestine. This likelihood seems most probably to be determined by the intraluminal environment rather than by mechanoreceptors, though the actual nature of the regulatory sensory mechanism remains to be described.

The program for the tonic contractions that define the haustral markings also remains completely unknown. It seems likely that it involves the same basic mechanisms for the generation of the tone that defines the sphincters of the gastrointestinal tract including the internal anal sphincter, but these mechanisms, probably strictly muscular mechanisms, are themselves not understood. Some very simple questions remain unanswered. For example, it is not clear whether the capacity of the colonic muscle to generate a haustral contraction is fixed, restricted to certain rings of muscle, or generalized, expressible at any point along the organ. If the latter case is true, what determines the uniform spacing of the contractions?

The defecation reflex, involving both the relaxation of the internal anal sphincter and a strong peristaltic contraction throughout the rectosigmoid segment, represents the action of the extrinsic innervation of the region. This effect represents a reflex involving a hypothetical defecation center that involves postulated centers in the spinal cord at the sacral level. The specific structures and operations of the defecation center have not even been seriously considered and so its nature remains conjectural. The defecation reflex appears to be initiated by sensory receptors, probably mechanoreceptors in the epithelium of the anal canal and possibly by other mechanoreceptors in the deeper layers of the rectal wall.

5.7.4. Colonic Flow

The entry of fluid into the cecum from the ileum is an intermittent or pulsatile event, a squirt, because ileal peristaltic contractions propel the fluid. Normally, the material remains in the cecum and the ascending colon for rather long periods because of the characteristic antiperistalsis of this part of the organ (see above). This retention allows time for the slow process of water absorption. Presumably, the physical or chemical characteristics of the cecal content govern the length of time that this process requires. That is, the conversion of the normal antiperistalsis into orthoperistalsis to empty the segment probably does not occur until the viscosity of the contained material has been changed by the extraction of a significant proportion of its water content. The movement of water across the membrane is passive, by diffusion.

The change in the direction of peristalsis might also depend upon changes in the chemistry of the luminal fluid, for a great deal of fermentation occurs here, the breakdown of undigested food elements, mainly complex carbohydrates, by the bacteria that inhabit the large intestine.

The long residence of the fecal mass in the rostral part of the large intestine permits the fermentation there of undigested or unabsorbed nutrients by fecal bacteria. A very large fraction of the mass of the feces excreted in defecation constitutes bacterial residues, and several hundred species of bacteria inhabit the large intestine. The organ can be considered a fermentation vat as well as a means to remove water from the fecal stream. In some species, notably many perissodactyls, the products of this fermentation are absorbed and contribute a large fraction of the energy supply for the animal. This is not true in man, however.

Within the major part of the large intestine, between the hepatic flexure and the rectosigmoid junction, the occlusive haustral markings divide the fluid intraluminal content into a series of pools. This effectively ends antegrade flow, allowing water absorption the time it needs. Since each haustral contraction can and often does effectively seal the lumen, the pockets they form are separate units in which the intraluminal pressure can become much higher than it would if the lumen remained open, allowing pressures to dissipate upstream or downstream. This fact is clearly important in understanding the pathogenesis of colonic diverticulosis (see Chapter 6).

At the infrequent intervals when the haustral markings disappear and a single peristaltic contraction occurs in the "mass movement", the contraction pushes the fecal mass a short distance antegrade, after which the haustral indentations recur. This event happens about three or four times daily so that the rectosigmoid part of the organ receives a mass of feces two or three times daily.

The rectosigmoid part of the large intestine seems to store these serial deliveries. The quanta of feces accumulate until a critical volume is achieved when the defecation reflex is excited. The consequent peristaltic contraction of the rectosigmoid then fully evacuates the fecal mass.

REFERENCES

[1] Christensen J. The Motility of the Colon. In: Johnson LR, Alpers DH, Christensen J, Jacobson ED, Walsh JH, Eds. Physiology of the Gastrointestinal Tract. 3rdedition. New York, Raven Press 1994; pp. 991-1024.

[2] Conklin JL, Christensen J. Motor Functions of the Pharynx and Esophagus. In: Johnson LR, Alpers DH, Christensen J, Jacobson ED, Walsh JH, Eds. Physiology of the Gastrointestinal tract. 3rdedition. New York, Raven Press 1994; pp. 903-928.

[3] Kelley KA. Motility of the Stomach and Gastroduodenal Junction. In: Johnson LR, Alpers DH, Christensen J, Jacobson ED, Walsh JH, Eds. Physiology of the Gastrointestinal Tract. 1stedition. New York, Raven Press 1981; pp. 393-410.

[4] Makhlouf G. Neuromuscular Function of the Small Intestine. In: Johnson LR, Alpers DH, Christensen J, Jacobson ED, Walsh JH, Eds. Physiology of the Gastrointestinal Tract. 3rdedition. New York, Raven Press 1994; pp. 977-990.

[5] Mayer E. The Physiology of Gastric Storage and Emptying. In: Johnson LR, Alpers DH, Christensen J, Jacobson ED, Walsh JH, Eds. Physiology of the Gastrointestinal Tract. 3rdedition. New York, Raven Press 1994; pp. 929-976.

[6] Meyer JH. Motility of the Stomach and Gastroduodenal Junction. In: Johnson LR, Alpers DH, Christensen J, Jacobson ED, Walsh JH, Eds. Physiology of the Gastrointestinal Tract. 2ndedition. New York, Raven Press 1987; pp. 613-630.

[7] Schulze K. Imaging and modeling of digestion in the stomach and the duodenum. Neurogastroenterol Motil 2006; 18: 172-183.

[8] Weisbrodt NW. Motility of the Small Intestine. In: Johnson Alpers DH, Christensen J, Jacobson ED, *et al*, Eds. Physiology of the Gastrointestinal Tract. 1stedition. New York, Raven Press 1981.

CHAPTER 6

Disordered Mechanical Function in the Gastrointestinal Tract

Abstract: This chapter evaluates disorders of regulatory mechanisms such as achalasia and Hirschsprung Disease and disorders of effector mechanisms such as reflux disease, systemic sclerosis of the GI tract and Colonic Diverticular Disease. Definitions, pathogenesis, course, treatment and complications are revealed as well as the bioengineering thoughts of the authors are elucidated.

Keywords: Achalasia, biomechanics, diverticular disease, gastroesophageal reflux disease, Hirschsprung Disease, motility.

6.1. INTRODUCTION

Proper function in the gastrointestinal tract requires that its mechanical operations be normal. Normal motor behavior in the gut, however, includes a good deal of variation because, as a self-regulated mechanical device, it monitors its own functions and modifies them continuously. Its scrutiny encompasses both mechanical events in relation to the physical conditions in the muscular wall and biochemical conditions in relation to the milieu of the gastrointestinal lumen. That is to say, neural mechanoreceptors in the gut wall and neural chemoreceptors in the gut mucosal epithelium receive a variety of kinds of inputs continuously and respond in ways that modify the mechanical functions of the gut.

Common usage often speaks of gastrointestinal diseases as disorders of absorption or secretion, or in terms of a morphological problem such as a cancer, an ulcer or a stone. Because the mechanical operation of the gut is so closely regulated by the mechanoreceptive and chemoreceptive inputs, disordered motor function occurs in most gastrointestinal diseases. Disturbed mechanical function is sometimes the most conspicuous aspect of the disease. The latter sort of clinical diseases are commonly spoken of as the motor disorders of the gut.

This chapter describes a few clinical states or diseases in which mechanical dysfunction is the major or apparently primary abnormality. They can be classified loosely as disorders chiefly of the mechanisms that regulate the contractions of the muscle and as disorders chiefly of the mechanisms that execute those motions. Basic reading about the diseases can be found in textbooks such as Sleisenger & Fordtran's Gastrointestinal and Liver Disease [1].

Hans Gregersen and James Christensen

These should be considered only as representative disorders, treated here from the perspective of biomechanics, not as an exhaustive list of the motor diseases of the gut. Our viewpoints presented in this chapter are based on clinical experience and common knowledge about these diseases. Our viewpoints on the selected diseases are also based on the biomechanical and bioengineerings ideas expressed in two key references by Gregersen [2, 3] as well as on the literature referred to in other chapters. Therefore, specific references are not provided in this chapter. The interested reader can easily find the relevant literature using literature databases.

6.2. DISORDERS OF REGULATORY MECHANISMS

6.2.1. Achalasia

6.2.1.1. Definition

The term, achalasia ("absent relaxation" in Greek), alludes to the failure of the esophagogastric sphincter to relax in swallowing as it normally does. A synonymous term, cardiospasm, implies that the force of contraction of that sphincter at rest is beyond the range of normal. Since this is not really the case, the latter term is being used less and less. Achalasia is defined by its typical pattern at manometry. The diagnosis can be supported by findings at barium radiography that may show delayed passage through the lower esophageal sphincter and dilatation of the body of the esophagus. At manometry, achalasia is characterized primarily by aperistalsis of the esophageal body and incomplete relaxation of the lower esophageal sphincter.

6.2.1.2. Gross Description

In achalasia, the striated muscle of the esophagus and that of the oropharynx function normally because extrinsic nerves regulate their operation, somatic nerve fibers that originate in the cranial nerve nuclei in the brainstem. As a result, the first stages of swallowing are normal.

The visceral muscle of the esophagus, however, responds abnormally to a swallow. Both the peristaltic contractions in the esophageal body (the part composed of visceral muscle) and the relaxations of the esophagogastric sphincter fail to occur normally. The tonic contraction of the esophagogastric sphincter that characterizes the resting state persists. As a consequence, swallowed material traverses the pharynx and upper part of the esophagus normally, arriving in a paralyzed organ segment, the caudal two-thirds of the esophagus, which tends to dilate because of the absence of the force needed to empty it and because the sphincter cannot relax. Only hydrostatic force can empty the contents of this part of the organ, so that only a small stream of fluid can ooze through the obstruction of the closed sphincter. At first, and for a long time, this hydrostatic force may overcome the sphincteric resistance adequately so that the obstruction is not complete and adequate nutrition is maintained, but the organ never really empties. Hydrostatic emptying progressively fails, however, and the organ becomes more dilated as time passes.

6.2.1.3. Course and Treatment

The disease often begins in young persons, and its dismal consequences, inadequate nutrition and chronic esophageal inflammation, demand treatment early in the diagnosis. The condition usually appears to be stable, but there is actually a progression in the degree of dilatation of the esophagus.

The only effective treatments available are those designed to reduce the degree of obstruction offered by the tonically contracted esophagogastric sphincter. The circular muscle layer in this structure can be ruptured either by forceful dilation of the segment with a balloon or by cutting it in a surgical intervention. Of course, such treatments also reduce the barrier the normal sphincter provides to gastroesophageal reflux, allowing the ingress of gastric contents into the esophagus and so enhancing esophageal inflammation.

6.2.1.4. Pathogenesis. Achalasia is an Acquired Disease of the Regulatory Mechanism

Mechanism in the smooth-muscled esophagus. The nerves in the intramural myenteric plexus in that organ deteriorate, possibly as the result of an autoimmune process, possibly as a consequence of a neurotropic virus infection or the effects of a neurotoxin. It seems likely that several different causes may exist, even though no one has ever been established. The disorder remains truly idiopathic in terms of its prime cause, at least for the form of the disease that occurs in Europe and North America.

In idiopathic achalasia, the dysfunction is always confined to the esophagus, a fact that is explained by the observation that the number of neurons in the myenteric plexus of the esophagus is normally much lower that the number found in other parts of her gastrointestinal tract. When a toxin attacks neurons of the myenteric plexus with equal intensity throughout the tract, a critical level will be achieved first in the esophagus because there are fewer there to begin with.

In Chagas' disease, a chronic infection with a trypanosome that is found in central and South America, achalasia develops along with megacolon as a late manifestation. The part of the colon affected, the most caudal extremity is also the part with the lowest density in distribution of nerve cells in the myenteric plexus. That form of achalasia is thought to be the consequence of an autoimmune process directed to the nerve cells that is initiated by the infection.

6.2.1.5. Complications

The disease itself interferes with nutrition, of course, and there is the risk of aspiration of esophageal content into the respiratory tract with a resultant pneumonia. Treatment reduces the likelihood of these complications, but it leads to another, the persistent reflux of gastric content into the esophagus.

Several physiological and mechanical mechanisms tend to oppose acid reflux into the esophagus (see Chapters I and V, and below). These mechanisms include:

- the high resting pressure in the lower esophageal sphincter
- the force of primary peristalsis
- the buckling of the mucosa and submucosa in the caudal part of the organ by the passive tension in the sphincteric muscle
- the presence and force of secondary peristalsis in the esophagus
- the flow of the buffering alkaline saliva through the esophagus
- the geometry of the esophagogastric junction and the esophageal hiatus, the esophagogastric angle
- the body posture during and after eating. After the breach of the sphincter in achalasia, the first four of these factors are gone

The first four mechanisms above are the most important. Two of them are absent in the treated patient with achalasia: the nerve damage has destroyed primary and secondary peristalsis and mechanical stretching or surgical incision has destroyed the barrier function of the lower esophageal sphincter and the mucosal buckling at that level produced by the compression of the sphincter.

The idea that the buckling of the mucosa in the distal esophagus is important as an opponent of reflux is rather new and untested. Whatever the magnitude of its effect may be in normal persons in this respect, it becomes more important when the disease and its treatment have removed the major factors opposing reflux. The cause of buckling, the passive tension of the muscle in the distal esophagus, presumably continues as long as the region does not become dilated. Dilation of the esophageal body as a consequence of the pooling in the region, however, must contribute to the reduction of the buckling. This speaks in favor of breaching the sphincter early in the course of the disease, as soon as the diagnosis is made, hoping to prevent the dilation of the esophageal body.

The further complications of gastroesophageal reflux are discussed later in this chapter.

6.2.1.6. Further Comments and Speculations

The assumption that the visceral muscle is normal in achalasia is not well supported. The fact that no lesions can be seen on routine histological examination does not exclude electron microscopic lesions. The usual histological methods show very little of the connective tissue in the organ and, in any case, cannot reveal anything about the functional or physical characteristics of the tissues. Indeed, one would reasonably expect some kind of physiological and structural change in a visceral muscle that is chronically denervated.

The idea that the primary damage occurs only to the intramural plexus of the esophagus is not fully supported. There was evidence long ago to suggest that the motor centers in the brainstem may be affected in some cases at least. In fact, there is a very limited amount of anatomic information about this matter.

The common idea that idiopathic achalasia, that not associated with Chagas' disease, is a single disease entity may not be true. Clinicians have long recognized "vigorous" achalasia as a special form with little dilatation of the organ and rhythmic spontaneous contractions in the musculature, as opposed to "classical" achalasia in which the muscle seems to be wholly inactive and the organ ultimately becomes greatly dilated. In "vigorous" achalasia, a form of the disease characterized by spontaneous non-peristaltic contractions of the visceral muscle segment, thickening of the circular muscle layer in the dysfunctional part of the organ has been noted. Also, some reports exist that the disease called esophageal spasm may evolve into achalasia, and there are rare reports of complete remission of achalasia.

The nerves that are destroyed or defective in achalasia seem to be the principal motor nerves of esophageal smooth muscle, nerves that act on the muscle by releasing nitric oxide. They normally account for both the relaxation of the sphincter and the peristaltic contraction of the esophageal body. They seem to be damaged simultaneously throughout the smooth muscle part of the organ, and so the mechanical failure occurs simultaneously in the sphincter and in the esophageal body. The characteristic dilatation of the esophageal body, however seems to develop and progress as a secondary change. The dilatation is, to a large degree, irreversible. Once it has taken place, it does not abate much when the obstruction is relieved by the breach of the obstructing lower esophageal sphincter. This may be the manifestation of a process of tissue remodeling. The dilatation is caused by the increased intraluminal content resulting in increased pressure and stretch of the wall. The outlet resistance and the aperistalsis are the causing factors. The wall in the esophageal body cannot contract properly and therefore gradually stretch. Most likely a turning point (from a therapeutic point of view) is when the esophagus lumen becomes wide open, that is when the buckling disappears due to the stretching. The intraluminal forces on the wall will be even bigger, resulting in more stretch. In addition when the wall is overstretched, it will be even more difficult for the muscles to make an efficient contractions. Such viewpoints are easy to understand with proper knowledge of even simple mechanical laws like Laplace's law.

Some sort of remodeling of the musculature undoubtedly takes place in a condition such as achalasia where the altered muscle function is permanent. For example, after breach of the sphincter by dilatation or cutting, the obstruction at this level may recur after a matter of several months or years. This can require repeated mechanical or surgical efforts to reduce the obstruction. There is essentially no information from morphological studies about the remodeling that must occur either as a result of the disease or as a result of the treatment. The use of the methods and concepts of bioengineering in the study of this matter might provide new ideas about the management of a disease in which the only useful treatment, breach of the lower esophageal sphincter, has remained essentially unchanged from the beginning of modern medicine.

6.2.2. Hirschsprung Disease

6.2.2.1. Definition

Hirschsprung disease also called congenital megacolon is a developmental disorder in which the newborn infant is observed to have a dilated colon.

6.2.2.2. Gross Description

The newborn infant, usually a male, shows infrequent or absent defecation with abdominal distension. The disease always involves the organ's caudal extremity, the internal anal sphincter, and a variable length of the colon above the sphincter. This whole segment remains tonically contracted, the unremitting contraction obstructing the flow of feces, and the colon rostral to the contracted segment becomes dilated.

6.2.2.3. Course and Treatment

In most infants, the obstruction is so complete that immediate treatment is necessary. Very rarely, the obstruction is of a lesser degree such that the infant grows into childhood, learning how to tolerate an irreversible disorder of defecation. In such cases, the degree of colonic distension can become truly astonishing.

Usually, however, Hirschsprung disease is treated promptly and definitively. The only treatment is the surgical removal of the contracted segment to relieve the obstruction. Various technical modifications in the surgical technique have not wholly compensated for the fact that it results in the absence or disturbed function of an internal anal sphincter postoperatively, and so lifelong disordered defecation, to a variable degree, plagues patients with this condition. After resection, the function of the colon rostral to the narrowed segment gradually returns to something like normal function.

6.2.2.4. Pathogenesis

The myenteric plexus in the contracted segment is abnormal with very few nerve cells and large contorted bundles of nerve fibers. The myenteric plexus in the dilated regions rostral to the contracted segment appear to be normal. This is now considered to be the consequence of a defective maturation of nerve cells in this region after they migrate here at a very early stage in embryogenesis. There is much speculation about the reason for this maturation disorder.

6.2.2.5. Complications

The principal complication of the disorder is the defective defecation that remains even after efforts have been made to preserve the internal anal sphincter. A degree of denervation in the region is inevitable, and sphincteric function is inevitable disturbed. Stricturing in the region is also not rare. The disorder seems never to affect other viscera.

6.2.2.6. Further Comments and Speculation

As in achalasia, some of the assumptions that are made about Hirschsprung disease lack the support of good evidence and some of the observations are unexplained.

The idea that the denervated muscle is itself otherwise normal rests on little good evidence. The routine histological examination reveals little or nothing about the connective tissue elements in the diseased segment, and it cannot provide any evidence at all about the physical properties of the tissue. It could well be that the muscle, being denervated from its first development, possesses distinctive physical properties as a result.

The view that Hirschsprung disease is a homogeneous disease entity finds little support from the considerable variability in the extent of the lesion and in the degree of functional difficulty that occurs. The underlying primary abnormality is not known. The variability that is seen in the disease could reflect simply variation in the length of the caudal part of the organ over which a single cause for defective maturation of the intramural nerves exerts itself. Alternatively, there could be two or more different causes for the maturation defect.

The idea that the rest of the colon above the obstructed segment is wholly normal is not established, even though it seems to function adequately after resection of the obstructing narrow segment. The considerations of the causes of the dilatation process are basically the same as those mentioned above for achalasia, perhaps with the difference that the colon is not collapsed and buckled like the esophagus. Since operation is normally done quite fast and in infants, it seems likely that the remnant colon can reverse towards normal function. This is somewhat in contrast to the irreversible condition in long lasting achalasia.

Remodeling must occur after treatment. Immediately after the surgical removal of the obstructing rectum or rectosigmoid, the remaining colon may possess abnormal mechanical properties, either as a residual of the disease itself or as a consequence of the operation. Biomechanical methods and concepts might illuminate this matter and so provide some guidance to the better management of the almost inevitable lifelong disordered defecation that plagues those who have had a distal colonic resection for Hirschsprung disease.

6.3. DISORDERS OF EFFECTOR MECHANISMS

6.3.1. Gastroesophageal Reflux Disease

6.3.1.1. Definition

The retrograde flow of the contents of the stomach into the esophagus damages the esophageal epithelium, sets up an inflammatory reaction there and leads to scar formation. The whole event, at any stage in its progression, constitutes the disease. It is often referred to by laymen as "heartburn", one of the common symptoms of early disease.

6.3.1.2. Gross Description

There are three fundamental processes operating in GERD, erosion, inflammation and repair.

When the injurious substances in the fluid contents of the stomach reach the esophageal epithelium, the damaged squamous cells at the surface peel off, thinning the epithelium and exposing deeper epithelial cells to the assault. This calls forth inflammatory cells which invade both the epithelium and the deeper layers of the esophageal wall. The epithelium may wholly disappear leaving esophageal ulceration. The inflammatory process initiates efforts at healing that include the deposition of connective tissue that is evident grossly as scarring.

Ulceration and scarring are most highly developed at the caudal extremity of the esophagus which is the most severely affected because that is where the noxious fluid enters the organ. The lesions diminish rostrally. Scarring is most evident in the formation of Schatzki's ring, a shelf of the mucosa that encircles the lumen at the junction of the esophageal to the gastric epithelium.

6.3.1.3. Course and Treatment

The process may begin at any age because of the many factors that contribute to it. Actually, a small degree of gastroesophageal reflux is normal at any age. It becomes pathological only when it exceeds a certain level in qualitative, quantitative or temporal terms. It ebbs and flows, partly as a result of intermittent treatment, but over a lifetime, it often seems to progress slowly but inexorably.

Treatment is aimed especially at suppression of the heartburn that is its chief symptom in its earlier stages. Other more rational treatments aim at reducing the noxious nature of the gastric content and increasing the mechanical factors that oppose reflux.

6.3.1.4. Pathogenesis

Hydrochloric acid, pepsin and bile salts, all constituents of the gastric juice, damage the esophageal epithelium when they enter the organ. They all would harm the gastric epithelium itself as well were there not mechanisms in that tissue to resist their noxious effects. As an organ of storage, the stomach also suffers from the potential for prolonged exposure to the potentially injurious agents found in many foods and drugs, but it seems also to be able to resist their effects to some degree.

The esophageal epithelium does not share the ability of the gastric epithelium to resist the destructive effects of the many injurious constituents of the gastric juice. As a result, some degree of damage to the esophageal epithelium frequently, if not always, accompanies gastroesophageal reflux, even if it is brief, and chronic reflux always produces extensive erosion, inflammation and repair.

The flow of the fluid contents of the stomach into the esophagus follows the gradient in global pressure between the abdomen and thorax. This gradient is normally opposed by the erect posture of humans. But other factors strongly affect the balance between those that foster reflux and those that oppose it.

The esophagogastric sphincter, described in Chapter 1, undoubtedly provides the principal barrier to gastroesophageal reflux and consequently the main defense against gastroesophageal reflux disease. It seems not to be perfect in its ability to prevent reflux, however, because probably everyone, including normal people, has experienced occasional heartburn, the immediate symptom produced when the nerves in the epithelium of the caudal part of the esophagus encounter gastric juice.

The relaxation of the sphincter that must occur in every swallow means that the resistance to flow through the junction is minimal for several seconds with each swallow, during a part of which time reflux can occur. If a little retrograde flow does take place during a swallow, the flow induced by the associated peristaltic contraction immediately sweeps the fluid back into the stomach, making such reflux inconsequential.

The important barrier function of this sphincter is the result of its tonic contraction at rest, between swallows, when it must oppose reflux throughout the whole array of occurrences that take place throughout the day and night, events that tend to favor gastroesophageal reflux by raising the intragastric pressure.

The force of this tonic contraction of the sphincteric muscle arises in large part from a special property of the muscle itself, involving a special metabolic system that remains obscure. The tonic contraction of the lower esophageal sphincter may well originate in a muscular specialization that characterizes all gastrointestinal muscles possessing tone and is most evident in those where tonic contraction is most prominent, the sphincters and the reservoirs (the gastric fundus and the cecum).

As well, the nerves that supply the muscle can modify this force, by increasing it or by lowering it, independent of the swallowing process. The sphincter seems to have the ability to raise the force of its own tonic contraction through the existence of mechanoreceptors that sense change in the pressure in the gastric lumen, probably through the detection of change in the strain in the gastric wall. The sphincter contracts as well with a rise in intraabdominal pressure, apparently as a response to mechanoreceptors in the surrounding muscles, perhaps in the diaphragm or the anterior abdominal wall. The mechanoreceptors in the viscera are still essentially purely theoretical constructs, having no structural or morphological identity, though they must activate a chain of linked sensory and motor nerves, a complete reflex pathway. The mechanoreceptors in the striated muscle, the muscle spindles, are well-known.

The failure of the esophagogastric sphincter to effectively overcome the gastroesophageal pressure gradient in all situations could represent a failure in the reflex regulation of the sphincter. As well, the failure of the sphincter in this respect could represent other influences that depress the ability of the muscle itself to exert its normal force in contracting. These factors are thought to include certain of the gastrointestinal hormones, the progestational hormones, and several substances in the diet. Empirical observation suggests that alcohol, coffee, chocolate, and mint flavoring all enhance gastroesophageal reflux by impairing the ability of the sphincter muscle to maintain a normal contractile force. The same is believed to be an effect of smoking tobacco, both acutely and chronically. In all these cases, the mechanism, the magnitude, and the duration of the effect can only be speculated about.

Esophageal peristalsis itself opposes reflux. When the peristaltic wave is initiated in eating, it must push back the any small amount of gastric content that entered the esophagus during the brief relaxation of the sphincter. When the noxious gastric fluid escapes through the esophagogastric junction at other times than those in a swallowing-induced relaxation of the sphincter, the fluid may set up a reflex that initiates a phenomenon called "secondary peristalsis". In this phenomenon, a peristaltic contraction that is not initiated by a swallow occurs in the smooth muscled part of the esophagus. The reflex seems to be supported by intrinsic nervous mechanisms alone. This event, not involving motions of the mouth or oropharynx and so being imperceptible, clears the distal esophagus of refluxed gastric juice. The reflex also operates to empty the esophagus when a small amount of swallowed food or a tablet of medicine is retained there, as often happens. Secondary peristalsis is thus an important normal reflex mechanism that operates to oppose reflux esophagitis.

The peristaltic wave, the front of contraction that moves as a ring through the organ after a swallow (primary peristalsis) or reflexly (secondary peristalsis), normally moves the whole content of the lumen into the stomach. It does this with a certain force that exhibits a vector in the antegrade direction. The magnitude of this force is clearly important is the effectiveness with which the process is carried out. If the force is diminished, clearance may be impaired. This force cannot be measured directly in the clinical situation, but it must reflect the magnitude of the contraction of the muscle. Hence, a reduction of the contraction force in the esophageal musculature must diminish the clearance of material from the organ. A diminished peristaltic contractile force can be both a cause and an effect of gastroesophageal reflux disease, making this a self-sustaining disorder.

Sometimes, the esophageal response to swallowing occurs not as a progressive contraction front but as a simultaneous contraction of the whole length of the esophageal body, often repetitive. Such non-propulsive or "simultaneous" contractions may come and go for no clear reason. Sometimes this sort of contraction does not appear uniformly along the length of the organ but at short intervals along the organ to create, for a moment, a chain of pockets in the organ. Such a pattern of contraction not only fails to clear the organ but retains refluxed gastric fluid in the organ, favoring the development or persistence of more serious stages in the disease.

The buffering action of salivary secretions also has an important place in the protection of the esophagus. Saliva, a mildly alkaline fluid, flows through the esophagus continuously as a result of the repeated swallowing that takes place unconsciously at times unrelated to eating and drinking. The volume varies throughout the diurnal cycle but it never ceases entirely. A very small amount of alkaline secretion also comes from the scattered submucosal glands in the esophagus.

The volume of saliva secreted per unit time declines gradually as a function of age and diminishes greatly in certain diseases, especially in diffuse systemic sclerosis and similar autoimmune diseases. In some such cases, gastroesophageal reflux disease constitutes a major problem of management, clearly representing the loss of the buffering effect of the saliva. In the autoimmune diseases, the force of contraction in the esophageal muscle is also diminished, so that the two mechanisms are complementary.

Intrathoracic pressures are always slightly lower than atmospheric pressure and much lower than intra-abdominal pressure. This constant hydrostatic differential favors the retrograde flow of gastric contents into the esophagus, but the effect is minimized or effectively overcome in man by the usual assumption of an upright posture, as in sitting and standing. Several obvious practices that favor the hydrostatic gastroesophageal gradient, such as prolonged recumbence and abdominal compression by garments or by bending over, seem in some cases to be significant in the pathogenesis of reflux esophagitis.

The geometry of the structures at the esophageal hiatus, the opening in the diaphragm through which the esophagus passes to reach the stomach, influences reflux. Several structural arrangements here have been thought to be of some significance in the prevention of gastroesophageal reflux, providing the opportunity for a set of extra-esophageal factors in the pathogenesis of reflux esophagitis. These factors are: the angle of His (the esophagogastric angle), the pinchcock action of the diaphragm, and the presence of herniation of the stomach through the diaphragm (hiatal hernia).

The Angle of His. The esophagus enters the stomach not end-on but at an angle, so that a crescentic fold of the stomach is interposed between the most caudal cm or two of the esophagus and the gastric fundus. One theory about the cause of reflux proposes that the stomach pushes this fold against the end of the esophagus and that the resulting lateral compression of the gastroesophageal junction is an important factor in opposing reflux. The restoration of this angle was once a major goal of operative interventions to treat chronic gastroesophageal reflux. The idea was largely abandoned after studies revealed that the degree of angulation between the esophagus and the stomach shows a poor correlation with the existence of reflux esophagitis.

The Pinchcock Action of the Diaphragm. The width of the esophageal hiatus in the diaphragm varies, and it was once proposed that a narrow hiatus importantly opposes gastroesophageal reflux by pinching the distal esophagus. This idea, too, once supported a goal of operative intervention in the treatment of reflux, to reconstruct the hiatus by bringing the edges of the hiatus closer together. Some support for the theory exists in the fact that the tonic contraction of the bands of diaphragmatic musculature adjacent to the hiatus disappears transiently with a swallow. This, however, does not establish the pinchcock action as a major factor and it currently gets little attention. It seems to be a minor factor in any case.

Herniation of the Stomach through the Diaphragm. The protrusion of a part of the stomach through the esophageal hiatus into the thorax is a very common anatomical abnormality, at least in Europe and North America. The strong association between such hiatus herniation and chronic reflux esophagitis long ago led to the idea that the herniation, by changing the normal structural relationship of the esophago-gastric junction to the diaphragm, destroys the barriers to gastroesophageal reflux. This concept supported or augmented the theories of the pinchcock action of the diaphragm and of the importance of the esophagogastric angulation.

Unfortunately, the surgical repair of these hernias, combined often with the restoration of the angle of His and the apposition of the edges of the hiatus to narrow it, did not satisfactorily relieve the reflux in all cases, and so such operations have been largely abandoned as a treatment for reflux esophagitis alone. This is not to say that hiatal herniation does not cause reflux esophagitis. Indeed, it seems likely that it does contribute to the disorder. The failure of the operations to cure the problem arose mostly from the high rate of recurrence of the hernia soon after the operation.

The herniation was once attributed to a raised intra-abdominal pressure, with no experimental evidence to support the idea. It is now clear that the herniation is a consequence of the fibrosis produced by the chronic inflammation in chronic gastroesophageal reflux. The shrinkage of the scar tissue formed in the esophageal musculature at the region where the inflammation is most intense (just above the esophagogastric junction) prevents the normal swallowing-induced relaxation of the longitudinal muscle layers at this level. Such relaxation normally prevents herniation of the stomach with esophageal shortening in swallowing. This scar transmits the force of the swallow-induced shortening of the rostral longitudinal musculature to the junction, drawing it up into the hiatus. As the hernia advances into the thorax, it ruptures the phrenoesophageal ligament and then becomes fixed in place. The resultant structural changes tend to maintain the reflux. Thus, hiatal herniation is a consequence of chronic reflux esophagitis and, once formed, sustains the basic pathologic process, reflux

6.3.1.5. Further Comments and Speculation

Gastroesophageal reflux disease is truly complex as evidenced by the many geometric, mechanical, and chemical factors mentioned above influencing the initiation and progress of the disease. Despite the numerous studies on the role of contractility of the stomach, the esophago-gastric junction, and the esophageal body, on mucosa permeability and other factors, the is still much to be learned about gastroesophageal reflux disease. Treatment strategy may be different paths from removing the acid source over surgery to endoscopic treatment. Many of these treatments seem rough in these times where individualized therapy is becoming more and more important. Even subtle geometric alterations or subtle changes in mechanical functions of the sphincter and esophageal body may led to reflux. Many individual geometric factors such as size, cross-sectional geometry, length, buckling pattern and interrelated mechanical factors such as muscle force (circumferential and axial), opening pressure, muscle length-tension properties, and viscoelasticity are undoubtedly important. We seem to lack optimal measurement methods and diagnostic tools to accurately detect the origin of the problem. By developing more comprehensive diagnostic batteries with optimized methods and if most patients will seek treatment in the health care system in due time, it should be possible to develop specialized and individual minimally evasive treatments, especially endoscopic treatments and surgeries, that has the wanted effect without significant side effects. Needless to say diagnostic and therapeutic schemes based on bioengineering and biomechanical skills, in addition to highly specialized clinical skills, are required for a successful outcome in the majority of patients.

6.3.2. Systemic Sclerosis (Scleroderma) of the Gut

6.3.2.1. Definition and Gross Description

Several seemingly related disorders share the pathological feature of gastrointestinal muscular fibrosis. They affect many different organs throughout the body, most conspicuously the skin which may become stiff, firm, taut and shiny. They also affect the gut, especially the esophagus where they induce the reflux esophagitis. Colonic function, pulmonary function and renal function all may be affected. The symptoms vary enormously according to the distribution of the disorder in the body.

6.3.2.2. Course, Pathogenesis, Complications and Treatment

These disorders, commoner in women, often begin in young adulthood and progress so slowly that the diagnosis is not made for years after onset. Thus, the effects of the altered mechanical properties of the gastrointestinal musculature can be, for a long time, so subtle and mild as to be dismissed as trivial or explained as the result of some aberrational dietary practice or an emotional disturbance.

The pathogenesis of these diseases in not clear. Most authorities consider them to be autoimmune in nature. The consequence of the fibrosis is a change in the mechanical properties of the gastrointestinal wall. The affected muscle layer loses the force of its contraction and becomes stiffened.

Patients suffering from systemic sclerosis have frequently clinical gastrointestinal manifestations, especially excessive deposition of collagen in the esophagus which may cause swallowing problems. As the organ most commonly and severely affected in scleroderma, the esophagus declares its involvement earlier that do other gastrointestinal viscera, in the form of chronic gastroesophageal reflux and reflux esophagitis in all its degrees of severity. The mechanical factors seem to develop simultaneously throughout the organ, so that a mild degree of esophageal enlargement or dilatation, a diminished force of the peristaltic contraction and a reduced force of the tonic contraction of the esophagogastric sphincter all occur at the same time. When the organ is examined visually, by radiography or at esophagoscopy, its stiffness may be quite obvious. Endoluminal US seems capable of defining morphologic as well as physiologic abnormalities of the esophagus in patients with scleroderma of the esophagus since it has been found that US images correlated with established pathologic descriptions like smooth muscle atrophy, variable fibrosis, and collagen deposition.

In addition to the mechanical changes in the esophagus that promote reflux esophagitis (the weakness of the peristaltic and sphincteric contractions), fibrosis of the salivary glands commonly occurs, diminishing the buffering effect of the saliva that normally counters the erosion of the esophageal epithelium by the gastric juice. Also, the inflammation itself promotes fibrosis in the esophagus, a scarring that is superimposed on the fibrosis that is a part of the disease process.

The fibrosis of visceral muscle that takes place in these diseases is usually less strongly expressed in the other gastrointestinal viscera. It can, however, produce such muscle weakness in the stomach as to impair gastric emptying and so lead to chronic nausea and vomiting with consequent nutritional compromise. When the pathological process affects the small intestine, the weakness of the peristaltic contractions allows the proliferation of bacteria in the lumen of that organ. The small intestine receives an abundance of bacteria in normal alimentation, and it prevents their overgrowth in the nutrient-laden medium of the intestinal lumen by passing them on to the colon before they have time to grow much. When this intestinal "housekeeper" function fails, the bacterial overgrowth impairs intestinal digestion and absorption, leading to a malabsorptive diarrhea. When the visceral muscle fibrosis affects the colon, its expected effect, constipation, is usually superseded by the volume of the fluid that the organ receives from the fibrotic small intestine, so that diarrhea prevails. The colon is usually the least affected of the gastrointestinal viscera in scleroderma.

6.3.2.3. Further Comments and Speculation

The treatment of the gastrointestinal involvement of systemic sclerosis as it affects the gut is the treatment of the conditions it induces there, gastroesophageal reflux disease in the case of the esophagus of bacterial overgrowth syndromes in the case of intestinal involvement.

From a bioengineering perspective with focus of the progressing dysfunction, the change in the matrix (the passive component) and the loss of muscle cells and muscle force (the active component) are two key factors. Though gastrointestinal physiology in a three-dimensional perspective is more complex than to be fully described by Hill′s model, then we can still learn from such models. The function or rather the remaining gastrointestinal function will inevitably depend on the interplay between the active and passive components.

6.3.3. Colonic Diverticular Disease (Diverticulosis Coli)

6.3.3.1. Definition and Gross Description

Multiple pockets, called diverticula, commonly in the wall of the large intestine. This condition is called diverticulosis. These diverticula may become infected. This is called diverticulitis.

The diverticula occur with special predilection for the sigmoid colon, the region just rostral to the rectum. However, occasional patients are seen to have them scattered more or less uniformly over most of the colon except for the cecum and rectum.

6.3.3.2. Course, Complications and Treatment

The occurrence of colonic diverticula seems clearly to be related to age. The condition is very rare in the first three decades of life but increases in incidence so that it is common in those past 60 years.

The condition is most often an incidental asymptomatic finding in persons examined appropriately for some other reason, but sometimes the diverticula themselves constitute the reason for the search, either because the are infected or because they bleed. Infection of diverticula can easily extend to become a life-threatening situation, and bleeding likewise can become the reason for emergency treatment. Infection, of course, is treated with antibiotics, but both infection and bleeding often requires surgical resection of the affected part of the organ, usually the sigmoid colon.

6.3.3.3. Pathogenesis

Diverticulosis clearly reflects a profound change in the mechanical properties of the colonic musculature but the reason for that change remains obscure. The change is manifest structurally as muscular hypertrophy, the cause of which remains unknown. Unfortunately good animal models of diverticulosis remain to be developed.

The hypertrophy develops first and becomes most severe in the sigmoid colon, the region just rostral to the rectum, and it can occur for a variable distance on toward the cecum. Only uncommonly does it occur in the colon above the hepatic flexure and it never occurs in the rectum.

Although the diverticula are the chief morphological manifestation of the smooth muscle hypertrophy, the hypertrophy antedates the appearance of the diverticula and it can be easily seen by any alert examiner. It appears to the radiographer and to the colonoscopist alike as indentations of the lumen by thick rings in the wall of the organ. At pathological examination, these indentations are clear as thick rings of the circular muscle layer. Appropriate studies have shown that they represent hypertrophy (an increase in muscle cell size) rather than hyperplasia (an increase in the number of muscle cells).

The parts of the large intestine in which the hypertrophy occurs manifest higher intraluminal pressures during the contractions that characterize colonic motor function than do the normal parts of the organ. This suggests that the diverticula are pockets pushed out by pathologically high intraluminal pressures.

As should be expected from the idea that the diverticula are pushed out, the diverticula form at the points of least resistance to distension in the colonic wall. These points are the sites at which the nutrient vessels to the colon penetrate the thickest layer of the wall, the circular muscle layer. At these spots, a knuckle of the mucosa is pushed through the opening in the layer of circular muscle, alongside the vessels, and protrudes to the outer surface of the organ, carrying over it the thin serosa.

The hypertrophy is confined to the circular muscle layer and the rings in which it occurs are widely separated. As a result, the contractions of these hypertrophied rings seal the lumen, dividing the organ into a series of separate compartments. The seal prevents the high pressures the abnormal muscle generates in these closed compartments from leaking into those parts of the colon that have been less affected by the hypertrophy.

Although modern teaching generally attributes the muscle hypertrophy to the lifelong adherence to a low-residue diet, convincing evidence and a rational explanation for that idea remains to be advanced. In physiological terms, the reason why such a diet should lead to such a change is obscure. However, animal models exist in rat and rabbit where low-residue diet are associated with the development of diverticula, 4-5 months diet in rabbits seems to induce diverticula as shown in studies back in the early seventies.

6.3.3.4. Further Comments and Speculation

The disease requires decades to become evident and this means that the hypertrophy probably begins its progress silently when its victims are still very young. Since the proximate cause is a change in the physical characteristics of the circular muscle layer of that region, the sigmoid colon, the detection of changes in the mechanical properties of the wall in that region in youth would be a predictor for the development of the disease in later life. It is widely believed, though contradicted recently) that the adherence to a low residue diet is the main causative factor in the hypertrophy, and patients with symptomatic diverticula are now instructed to adhere to a diet high in residue. If the condition could be detected at a much earlier stage, this dietary change could perhaps be made at a time when it would have the effect of preventing the progression of the diverticula.

This disease raises the broader question of the origin of hypertrophy in visceral muscle. A bioengineer with skills in biomechanics would have no doubt that this is a mechanical problem, based on the increased pressure and stresses in the tissue causing the weak points to yield. Much is however to be learned. One may ask why our knowledge of this disease is so little when it is so frequent. The explanations can probably be found in the fact that diverticulosis by itself is symptom-less, it develops over many years blurring the cause-response association, good animal models of diverticulosis do not exist and only few have an interdisciplinary approach to the problem.

6.4 SOME BIOENGINEERING THOUGHTS ABOUT THE MOTOR DISORDERS OF THE GASTROINTESTINAL TRACT

A consideration of these clinical states and the bioengineering approach outlined in chapter 2 reveals how little structured information is available on the biomechanics of disease in the motor apparatus of the gut. Rather we have only scattered bits of information, often the result of empirical observations made without a theoretical basis. For none of the diseases of this kind do we have the necessary information for a detailed understanding of the morphology, the anatomy, the structure and composition of the tissue and for the basic biophysical properties of the tissues.

The inaccessibility of organs and the unavailability of tissues in many patients with motor diseases (and in normal persons), make the modern investigator turn to the methods of physical modeling and mathematical modeling (or numerical simulation) to examine properly the physical processes that operate in gastrointestinal motility. Valid modeling and simulation, however, require valid data that can only be obtained from real tissues and experiments. When real tissues are not available from humans, we seek the basic information we need from animals. This may be reasonable because, at the most fundamental level, the constitutive equations for soft tissues may not differ much among species or even among organs. However, the material constants will likely differ to an important degree among species and organs, but methods such as those outlined in this book are becoming available for the mechanical testing of the gastrointestinal tract *in vivo*. Hence, material constants can be obtained in humans.

The advances that are mentioned in this book can do much to alter our management of motor dysfunction in the gastrointestinal tract in the future. They include especially the method that combines distension of an intraluminal bag with the depiction of the tension-strain relationship *in vivo*, the advances in medical imaging and 3D-modeling, and the development of new theory to combine data on the properties of tissues and fluid flow. They all can advance our knowledge if they are properly applied. This will require, however, a general appreciation for and understanding of mechanics on the part of all who think seriously about disorders of this kind. The need, then, is for training and education as well as for methods and concepts, and especially for collaboration between those two camps, the engineers who know about material behavior and the biologists and physicians who understand the behavior of tissues and of patients. The selected diaseases described earlier in this chapter are all of huge clinical interest as well as they are complex if the viewing eyer are clinical eyes only.

They represent a variety of conditions with different components of the organ system and behavior being affected. An interdisciplinary approach is needed for understanding and differentiation of the various components influencing the disease development.

REFERENCES

[1] Sleisenger & Fordtran's Gastrointestinal and Liver Disease: Pathophysiology, Diagnosis, Management. Eds. Feldman M, Friedman LS, Brandt LJ. 8th edition. Saunders 2006.

[2] Gregersen H. Biomechanics of the Gastrointestinal Tract. Springer Verlag, London. 2002.

[3] Gregersen H, Kassab GS. Biomechanics of the Gastrointestinal Tract. Neurogastroenterology and Motility 1996; 8: 277-297.

Clinical Mechanics in the Gut
An Introduction

CHAPTER 7

Future Perspectives

Abstract: To many physicians, gastrointestinal mechanics often seems a matter of pipes and valves. To gastrointestinal physiologists, gastrointestinal mechanics seems hugely complicated and still, to a large degree, incomprehensible. Most engineers probably have thought so little about the matter to have any opinion about it at all.

7.1. THE OUTLOOK FOR THE PHYSICIAN

The ignorance and widespread neglect of the evidence that exists on gastrointestinal mechanics belies the fact that gastrointestinal diseases are ubiquitous and bring about much disability and death. Disordered gastrointestinal motor function is a part of most gastrointestinal disease. It constitutes the major problem in esophageal disease, in diverticulosis of the colon, and in such rare conditions as the syndromes of intestinal pseudo-obstruction. Many people blame abnormal motor function for the irritable bowel syndrome. Also, motor disorders frequently complicate long-standing diabetes, several connective tissue diseases, and many neurological disorders. The prevalence and persistence of such clinical problems leave a large population of chronically ill people facing the consequences of defective gastrointestinal functions.

In respect to disease, we have very little structured information on the biomechanics of the motor apparatus of the gut. The scattered bits of information that exist about gastrointestinal mechanics in pathological conditions are often the result of empirical observations made without a theoretical basis. Consider the eight basic points put forth in Chapter 2 as the heart of the bioengineer's approach to any biomechanical system. For none of the known diseases of this kind do we have the necessary information for even the first two requirements: A detailed understanding of the morphology, the anatomy, the structure and composition of the tissue (point 1) and information about the basic biophysical properties of the tissues (point 2).

The application of the science of biomechanics to clinical problems in gastroenterology can be expected to do as much for the practice as it has already done for the practice in cardiovascular disease and orthopedics. Of course, the enormous complexity of the gastrointestinal tract makes it clear that the utility of biomechanics will be much slower in coming than in those other clinical disciplines. However, much can be done immediately. Methods already exist, relying on valid concepts, which could do much to alter our management of motor dysfunction in the gastrointestinal tract. We see especially the need for the application of the method that combines balloon distension with the depiction of the tension-strain relationship *in vivo.* Improved medical imaging and 3D-modeling and the development of new theory to combine data on the mechanical properties of tissues and fluid flow can also greatly advance our knowledge if they are properly applied.

7.2. THE OUTLOOK FOR THE GASTROINTESTINAL SCIENTIST

Of course, the rational management of the motor disorders of the gut, as in all aspects of medicine, requires accurate knowledge of pathophysiology, and that can come only from knowledge of the science of physiology. In the same way, the science of physiology can grow only from the correct uses of the physical sciences, physics and chemistry [1].

Although the history of the study of gastrointestinal mechanics is very long, it was shallow until the past half-century, and much of what has been done in the recent flowering of research has used methods and concepts of the century before, established by the study of other physiological systems.

The approach of recent gastrointestinal physiologists to the motor functions of the system seemed anachronous to biologists working at "the cutting edge" with techniques like those of molecular biology. It was necessary, however, to use old-fashioned methods in order to bring the knowledge of gastrointestinal science into the 20th century. We had to tie bits of thread on to the ends of muscle strips, we had to look at tissues with the light microscope, and we had to drop drugs into muscle baths, because such simple methods were necessary to learn the simple thing we did not yet know. Now, at last, one can begin to describe gastrointestinal motor functions in terms of concepts consistent with our understanding of contemporary neurobiology, modern visceral muscle structure and function, membrane transport, electrophysiology, and so on.

One cannot, however, describe the motions, the mechanics, of the various gastrointestinal organs in such a clear way as one can describe blood flow and the operation of the heart and the vasculature. It remains for mechanics to apply itself to the gut in the interest of gastrointestinal science.

Our knowledge of the mechanical function of the normal gastrointestinal tract remains sparse and unstructured, and we still lack adequate descriptions of many basic processes. Everyone who described mechanical behaviors in the gut in the past attempted to analyze or explain them, but their explanations failed often to pass the first tests for truth, the consistency of the explanations with known anatomy and physiology. Sometimes, the explanations offered even contravened principles of bioengineering and the physical laws!

In such a situation, the ability to predict behavior under prescribed normal circumstances vanishes. Surely, the test of any concept in physiology is the demonstration of its ability to predict the effect of altered circumstances on the operations of the system under consideration. The fact that we cannot do this with respect to the motions of the gastrointestinal tract simply reflects the fact that the system, despite all the advances of recent years, remains essentially a matter of considerable mystery.

We have long known of the adaptability, the plasticity, of the gastrointestinal tract. It can change remarkably in response to operative removal or modification of various organs or parts of organs, for example. Over the years, many important observations have been made about this process, including the alteration that various conditions can produce in intestinal structure, motor activities, cell morphology, metabolism, cell kinetics, and growth-regulating factors. However, many aspects of gastrointestinal adaptation are still not clear or even wait to be specified, and the mechanisms involved in generating these changes remain largely obscure. Biomechanics may well have an important role in the mechanisms of physical remodeling in response to environmental changes. A better description of the biomechanical properties that dictate the nature of remodeling is an important step in the exploration of the intestinal adaptation.

Among several other issues, further studies are needed to address such problems as the neural "mechanoreceptors" and "nociceptors" postulated on evidentiary grounds but still undefined in structural terms. The relationship between mechanoreceptors and nociceptors remains obscure. There are very likely several different kinds of mechanoreceptors. The analysis of the excitation of mechanoreceptors requires the application of biomechanics. A better knowledge of mechanoreceptors will benefit our understanding of how self-regulation works in the gut. It should also clarify the mechanisms involved in intestinal adaptation, in repair after injury, and in the perception of gastrointestinal events.

7.3. THE OUTLOOK FOR THE BIOENGINEER

The engineer who is interested principally in ways to alter the physical world in order to accomplish some human goal, must marvel at the way the gastrointestinal tract has been designed to accomplish its purposes. The mechanisms operating in the gut challenge comprehension at the most fundamental level partly because we lack data and partly because the system is so complicated. Even the basic process that occurs in the small intestine, axisymmetric peristaltic pumping all along a long conduit, with its exemplary efficiency, still defies adequate mathematical description and analysis.

Engineering represents the application of the principles of physics to the examination of physical processes, and bioengineering constitutes the application of such principles to biological processes. Now, we are on the verge of having the ability to make such an application in this particular area because of the progress we can foresee in the investigation, by mechanical means, of the specific motor performances of the various gastrointestinal organs. However, an old problem in biology persists in this area, which the behavior may change under the conditions necessary for its observation. The gut is hard to get at, and it is so sensitive that instruments designed to reveal its mechanical functions almost certainly change those functions.

The inaccessibility and behavioral inconstancy of the gut, as well as the increasing unavailability of tissues, make the modern investigator turn to examine the possible use of the methods of physical modeling and mathematical modeling (or numerical simulation) to examine properly the physical processes that operate in normal and disordered gastrointestinal motility. Valid modeling and simulation, however, require valid data that can be obtained only from actual tissues. When human tissues are not available, we seek the basic information we need from animals. This may actually be a reasonable approach because, at the most fundamental level, the constitutive equations for soft tissues may not differ greatly among species or even among organs. However, the material constants may well differ to an important degree among species and organs. Methods such as those outlined in this book are becoming available for the mechanical testing of the gastrointestinal tract in vivo so that material constants can now be obtained in humans.

Proper constitutive equations for the gastrointestinal tract are very much needed. Once the constitutive equation is known, the distribution of physical stresses and strains in the duodenum *in vivo*, and the functions of bolus transport and fluid movement in the gastrointestinal tract can be analyzed by the methods of continuum mechanics. The analytical results will relate the stress and function with the geometric parameters of the anatomy. Determination of the constitutive equations is not as big a task as might be expected because the mathematical form of most soft tissues is known. If it can be verified that the constitutive equations of the gastrointestinal tissues are similar to those of other soft tissues, then the principal task remaining is to determine the material constants of the gastrointestinal tissues with the instruments currently being developed for accomplishing this goal.

As pointed out previously, each organ exhibits specialization in a shared basic structure and regulatory system in order to accomplish the specific function it has in the body economy. The benefit of the imitation of nature in the design of machines has been clear for a very long time. The study of the unique pumps of the gut similarly might guide engineers who wish to design machines to do similar work. Such a study is prerequisite to imitation.

Major progress, however, requires a two-way communication. Those biologists who know the alimentary canal need to gain a proper appreciation for and understanding of the science of mechanics. And engineers need to have biologists to show them what they know, or how they see things.

The need, then, is for broader training and education as well as for new methods and concepts. And most important, there must be constant interchange and collaboration between two camps, the engineers who truly know about material behavior and those biologists and physicians who understand in part and wonder in part at the mechanical behavior of the gastrointestinal tract.

REFERENCES

[1] Christensen J. History of the evolution of ideas in gastrointestinal motility. In: Kirsner JB, Eds. The growth of gastroenterologic knowledge during the twentieth century. Philadelphia, Baltimore, Hong Kong, London, Munich, Sydney, Tokyo, Lea & Febiger 1994; pp. 140-59.

Clinical Mechanics in the Gut
An Introduction

Subject Index

A

B

C

D

E

Hans Gregersen and James Christensen

F

G

H

T

U

V

W

Made in the USA
Las Vegas, NV
03 November 2026

57425095R00152